MAN'S ENVIRONMENTAL PREDICAMENT

D. F. OWEN

Man's Environmental Predicament

AN INTRODUCTION TO
HUMAN ECOLOGY IN TROPICAL AFRICA

OXFORD UNIVERSITY PRESS

LONDON   OXFORD   NEW YORK

1973

Oxford University Press

OXFORD LONDON NEW YORK

GLASGOW TORONTO MELBOURNE WELLINGTON

CAPE TOWN IBADAN NAIROBI DAR ES SALAAM LUSAKA ADDIS ABABA

DELHI BOMBAY CALCUTTA MADRAS KARACHI LAHORE DACCA

KUALA LUMPUR SINGAPORE HONG KONG TOKYO

Hardbound edition ISBN 0 19 215650 0
Paperback edition ISBN 0 19 285062 8

© *Oxford University Press 1973*

*First published simultaneously in hardbound form and as an Oxford University Press
paperback 1973*

*Printed in Great Britain by
Richard Clay (The Chaucer Press), Ltd.,
Bungay, Suffolk*

PREFACE

Ecology is the study of the relationships between organisms and their environment. Man is an organism and the ecology of man can be studied like that of any other organism. Human ecology is therefore an attempt to examine man in relation to the environment. This is what I have tried to do in this book, picking tropical Africa as the environment because it seems to me that here some of the most rapid environmental changes that have ever occurred on earth are now taking place.

The state of the environment is becoming an important political issue in the economically developed countries of the world, and for the first time in history ecologists are finding themselves in the curious position of being regarded as the only people who can supposedly make valid judgements about the present state and future prospects of the environment. Unfortunately few ecologists can make sensible predictions about what will happen, except that the situation is rapidly growing worse and in some parts of the world it is already intolerable. There is of course only one real problem: rising human numbers and expanding human demands on the limited resources of the world. All other problems stem from this and all efforts at development are sooner or later thwarted by the number of mouths that have to be fed.

There are numerous books on the problems of economic development in tropical Africa, but they do not take into account the biological consequences of development proposals. I have tried to fill the gap with this book. In doing so I have read large numbers of scientific papers and books and some of these are cited as references. I estimate that I have cited about 10 per cent of what I have read and that I have read only about 1 per cent of what is available. There is a vast literature which has a bearing on Africa's ecological predicament, and it is scattered through medical, agricultural, sociological, political, and biological journals. My own experience in reading and travelling is largely confined to English-speaking Africa, but I have had the benefit of working for extended periods at two African universities, in Uganda and in Sierra Leone, and have thus come into contact with people in all walks of life: peasant cultivators, international experts in development and education, students, academics, and politicians. This experience has, I hope, been of some use in trying to interpret the findings in the literature, but I am aware that much of what I have to say is incomplete. Thus I have not cited the excellent work in French which is mainly about the French-speaking nations of tropical Africa. I have omitted Madagascar, and in restricting myself to tropical Africa I have not felt obliged to discuss in detail the peculiar situation that has developed in South Africa. Neither have I considered North Africa which is ethnically and biologically distinct from tropical Africa.

The book is intended as an introduction to the ecology of man in tropical Africa and in writing it I have tried to consider man as an ecologist might consider any other organism. The basic requirements of man are the same as those of other organisms, and although man may attribute special properties to himself which he believes set him apart from other animals, it is possible to place man in an ecological setting and to examine his interactions with the environment. I hope that what I have written will be useful not only to biologists interested in human ecology, but also to economists and sociologists, and to people who simply want to know something about the biological background to economic development in tropical Africa. I must also add that I would be the last to propose dogmatic solutions to Africa's ecological predicament. I firmly believe that attempts to solve the numerous problems that have been created must come from within Africa itself: a peasant farmer in Mali has just as much right to determine his destiny as a business man in London has to determine his.

Finally, I should point out that Chapter 10, which is about natural selection and genetics, is something of a digression from the main theme of the book. It is the only chapter which might be difficult reading for a non-biologist, but it can be skipped; and anyone with an elementary knowledge of genetics will have no difficulty.

D. F. OWEN

CONTENTS

LIST OF PLATES

LIST OF TEXT FIGURES

ACKNOWLEDGEMENTS

We should like to acknowledge the following for permission to use photographs: the *Guardian* for Plate 1; Ministry of Information, Uganda, for Plate 2; Professor T. L. Green for Plate 3; Jennifer Owen for Plates 4, 5, 6, 7, 10, 11, 14, 16; The Pyrethrum Bureau, Kenya, for Plates 8 and 9; The Centre for Overseas Pest Research for Plates 12 (C. Ashall) and 13 (J. Roffey and E. S. Brown); and The Inter-University Council for Higher Education Overseas, London, for Plate 15.

CHAPTER 1

The Environment and the People

The area under consideration in this book covers about 20 million km² of Africa between the Tropics of Cancer and Capricorn. But I have not been too rigid in this definition and there are some references to situations outside the area, especially in the south of the continent. Fig. 1 shows the present political divisions of tropical Africa and Table 1[1] the area of each country. To the north, tropical Africa is separated from the Mediterranean region by the Sahara Desert, the largest desert in the world, while to the east and west the sea forms a boundary. The southern third of Africa changes gradually and in the extreme south the environment is reminiscent of that of the Mediterranean region.

Tropical Africa is ecologically a diverse area, but two major components dominate: the forest and the savanna. Throughout this book the ecology of these two environments will be contrasted. Within tropical Africa, especially in the east, there are mountains rising to 6000 m and enormous freshwater lakes, including Lake Victoria, the second largest lake in the world. With the exception of the Nile, which flows northwards to the Mediterranean, most of the larger rivers enter the Atlantic. The Rift Valley cuts through the eastern part of the continent and many of the highest mountains of East Africa are associated with its formation.

The climate varies markedly from place to place, the most conspicuous variations being associated with altitude. Because much of East Africa is above 1500 m the climate is cooler than in the west and, except on the slopes of the larger mountains, considerably drier. Throughout much of lowland tropical Africa the temperature remains relatively constant all year and daily fluctuations are greater than seasonal ones. In the humid (forested) parts of this area the temperature rarely exceeds 35° C and rarely falls below 18° C.

[1] Tables are gathered at the end (pp. 188–98). They are not essential but are provided as an elaboration of certain points made in the text.

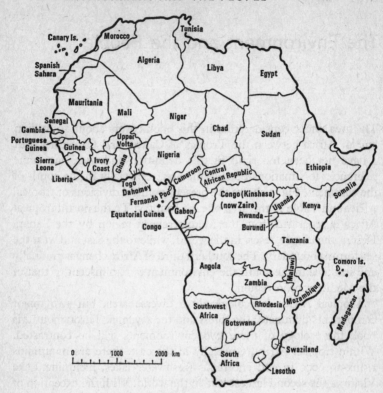

Fig. 1 Political map of Africa.

Frost does not occur except high on mountains. In the more arid savanna, temperature changes are more marked and at times it can become distinctly cool, especially north of the equator when in the dry season the wind blows from the Sahara. Coastal West Africa is extremely humid and relative humidities of 100 per cent are frequently recorded, even at the times of year when rainfall is slight.

The amount and seasonal distribution of rainfall are the most important climatic factors affecting plant and animal life in tropical Africa, and in many ways rainfall takes the place of temperature which at high latitudes is of greater importance. In nearly all areas rainfall is seasonal, and there may be one or two rainy seasons in a year alternating with periods of relative drought. The rainfall occurs more uniformly throughout the year and in greater amounts in the humid coastal areas of West Africa, and in some places the annual total may reach 400 cm. Seasonal rainfall dominates the lives of most of the people as it determines their activity in terms of planting and harvesting the crops, and of the movements of cattle and other domestic animals. But much of Africa is relatively arid, and the conditions in the savanna can become extremely harsh towards the end of the dry season. There is evidence suggesting that the impact

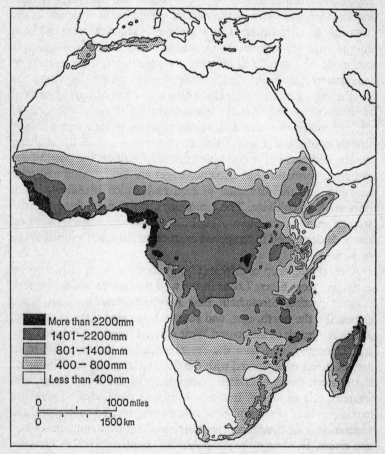

More than 2200mm
1401–2200mm
801–1400mm
400 – 800mm
Less than 400mm

0   1000 miles
0   1500 km

Fig. 2 Mean annual rainfall in Africa.

of man on the landscape has relatively recently reduced the biological effectiveness of rainfall, especially in areas where the savanna borders the desert, by increasing the evaporation rate. Indeed some people feel that Africa is rapidly drying up and have become concerned at the consequences of this for human welfare. Fig. 2 is a very much simplified map showing the mean annual rainfall in Africa.

The soil cover of Africa is variable. Vast areas are covered with laterite, a hard rocky substance formed when mineral-rich earth is exposed to sun and rain. This process, called laterization, is increasing as more and more of the natural vegetation is removed in the interests of cultivation. There are now extensive areas of hard laterite that are impossible to cultivate and it seems that man's continued attempts at cultivation are speeding up the process of laterization (McNeil, 1964). Soils develop primarily from the weathering of rocks, but include also quantities of humus derived from decomposing organic matter, chiefly plants. The rate of decomposition in warm and humid climates is high which means that most of the nutrients in an ecosystem are locked up in living plants. Removal of the vegetation not only removes the possibilities of humus formation but also encourages erosion by wind and rain, leaching, and the formation of hard rock which is difficult if not impossible to cultivate. These processes, which are a feature of the tropics throughout the world, help to explain why agricultural methods developed in temperate areas often fail when applied in the tropics.

A vegetation map of Africa (Fig. 3) shows an area of rain forest extending from Sierra Leone in the west to Uganda in the east with isolated patches throughout East Africa, especially on mountain slopes. To the north, east, and south of this area there is savanna. There is a break in the coastal West African forest in Ghana, Togo, and Dahomey, and here the savanna reaches the sea. The main area of forest is associated with the Congo River and its tributaries, the western forest of Sierra Leone, Liberia, the Ivory Coast, and western Ghana being isolated from the remainder. There are extensive areas of swamp, especially in the east and centre, and the vegetation is of course considerably modified by mountains, lakes, and rivers. In some quite small African countries, such as Uganda, variations in altitude result in an almost complete spectrum of world vegetation types: semi-desert in the north, rain forest around the shores of Lake Victoria, montane vegetation on the slopes of mountains, and permanent snow and ice on the tops of high mountains like Ruwenzori.

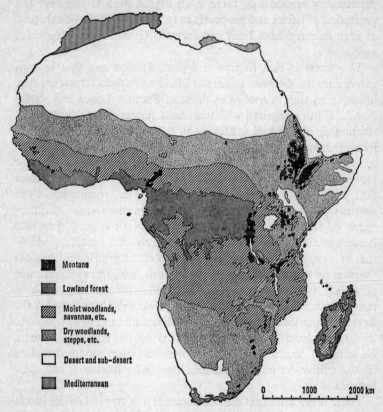

Montane

Lowland forest

Moist woodlands, savannas, etc.

Dry woodlands, steppe, etc.

Desert and sub-desert

Mediterranean

0   1000   2000 km

Fig. 3 Vegetation map of Africa.

The vegetation maps are, however, misleading because almost everywhere man has altered the natural cover of plants either by cultivating or by grazing domestic animals. Much of the forest area of Africa is now secondary bush, consisting of a complex mixture of the original forest vegetation, introduced crops and their weeds, and elements of the savanna vegetation that have colonized after the forest has been partially or completely cleared. A similar process has occurred in the savanna where, as already mentioned, the most conspicuous effect is the drying up of the landscape, encouraged no doubt by dry season grass fires started by man. It has been persuasively argued that there is an urgent need to conserve the vegetation of Africa and proposals as to how this might be achieved in each country have been put forward (Hedberg and Hedberg, 1968).

The forest is rich in tree and plant species and this in turn determines the diversity of animal life. The African forests are not, however, as rich in species as those of South America and southeast Asia, but compared with temperate forests their complexity is astounding and indeed confusing to the ecologist. In undisturbed forest there is little grass and most of the woody vegetation consists of saplings of the same species as the larger trees. Most of these saplings can only develop to maturity when one of the larger trees falls down and a vacant space is created. The topography of the savanna varies in different parts of Africa, partly because of differences in climate, especially in the amount of rainfall, but also because of differences in soil. The savanna environment is essentially that of a grassy plain or park, with trees either growing fairly close together or well spaced at regular intervals, and often with clumps of woody vegetation that are associated with the dispersion of termite mounds. There is of course no clear boundary between the forest and the savanna and such boundaries that might have existed in the past have been largely obscured by the activities of man. In terms of human ecology the forest has been modified mainly by the cultivators and the savanna mainly by herdsmen and their animals.

There is evidence that the rain forest belt of tropical Africa has in the past been both larger and smaller than it is now. In the past 100 000 years areas of forest have repeatedly been fragmented from one another and then joined again as the climate changed. During the past million years there were a series of glaciations that affected most of the northern hemisphere, especially at high latitudes. These glaciations undoubtedly exerted changes on the climate and vegetation of tropical Africa. A few degrees fall in temperature can increase the biological effectiveness of rainfall by reducing the evaporation rate, and under these conditions one would expect the vegetation to become more lush. As recently as about 10 000 years ago much of the Sahara was covered with vegetation and supported a considerable diversity of animal life, but with the slight rise in temperature that has occurred since then, the vegetation has largely disappeared and is still disappearing from around the edge of the desert, especially now that man is exerting such an influence upon it. It was probably the drying up of the Sahara that forced herdsmen to move south into the northern savannas of tropical Africa and it would also seem likely that this is how cultivation first arrived in the area. Space does not permit a detailed analysis of the past climatic and vegetational changes that have occurred in Africa; these have been competently reviewed elsewhere, notably by Moreau (1966). There is however no doubt that climatic changes have profoundly affected the ecology of man in tropical Africa and also man's cultural and physical evolution.

Evidence is rapidly accumulating that ape-men and man-apes passed through a succession of evolutionary changes in eastern and southern Africa and that these changes were in one way or another associated with changes in the climate. It is not my intention to discuss the fossil history of man as this can be found in specialized publications on the subject and in almost any biology text book. It is not known if the species we call *Homo sapiens* originated in Africa although it is known that many of the evolutionary changes leading to *Homo sapiens* occurred there, including, as well as the development of distinctive anatomical features, the use of tools and, especially, the use of weapons.

Animals and plants are classified into species. In sexually reproducing organisms species are defined as groups of interbreeding individuals that are unable to breed with individuals of other groups. Many species of animals are divided up into geographical subspecies and are designated as such by a trinomial. It is not the custom to do this for man even though it is obvious that man is geographically variable. The term race is synonymous in biology with the term subspecies, but it has received other rather loosely applied meanings in anthropology. There are, however, three main geographical groups of people, the negroids, caucasoids, and mongoloids, which are biologically equivalent to the races or subspecies of other organisms, and the fact that they have not been formally named does not mean that they do not exist.

The word tribe is used in animal classification as a taxonomic group lying between the genus and the family. The term is not in wide use and many groups are not classified according to tribe. But in man the word tribe has come to have a rather different and extremely ambiguous meaning. It is often used to denote a group, defined in terms of culture and physical appearance, that exists within what could be called the subspecies. Thus the Yoruba of Nigeria are a tribe[1] and so are the Baganda of Uganda, but within each there are numerous smaller units which, for want of a better term, are spoken of as ethnic groups. In biological terms these would be roughly equivalent to populations, a population being defined as a group of freely interbreeding organisms within a species which is geographically and ecologically isolated from other populations. Populations of organisms thus differ from each other in the occurrence and frequency of certain genes, and they remain distinct essentially because they are isolated by geographical and ecological barriers. Thus for a population of land snails a road may be a major ecological barrier to the dispersal of genes from one population to another and so it is possible for there to be two populations one on either side of the road. It appears that similar barriers can occur between human populations, but reinforced by cultural and religious differences. Cultural and religious barriers may become so strong that they replace geographical and ecological ones; consequently, unlike other animals, different populations of man can live together, as in a town, yet remain discrete. Hence biological populations in man are often referred to as ethnic groups, but unfortunately the term is used loosely, and it is not always clear what an anthropologist or sociologist means when he refers to an ethnic group. The term nation has no biological meaning and in Africa it has little ethnic meaning either, as the present nations frequently include people of diverse ethnic origin. Andreski (1968) has attempted to define these various concepts from the sociological point of view, and he admits that there are serious difficulties. He

---

[1] Anthropologists sometimes speak of the Yoruba and other large groups as a 'people'. The word 'tribe' is often restricted to mean the maximal political unit: this is certainly a valid definition, but it is not of great value in a biological sense.

suggests that social aggregates that are frequently referred to as tribes might be called 'ethnies' (singular 'ethny') which is a word now used in French.

It is a pity that no suitable terminology seems to exist that takes into account both the biological and cultural variations in man. There would in fact be no great difficulty in splitting man into three subspecies, acknowledging that (as with all subspecies) there are intergrades, and from then on speaking simply of populations, indicating as one does so the amount of genetic and cultural similarity and difference that exists between the populations. In this book I have so far as possible avoided the use of the word tribe, although I often use the name commonly given to a group of people, and whenever I use the term ethnic group I am in essence talking of what a biologist would call a population.

Much publicity has been given to discoveries in East and South Africa of fossil ape-men, but these fossils are too old and too different from modern man to throw light on the origin of the negroids, at present the most numerous people in tropical Africa. Indeed the origin of the negroids is obscure, far less being known about them than the other two major types of man, the caucasoids and the mongoloids.

Negroids have dark skins, curly woolly hair on the head, and little hair on the body. The lips are strongly everted, the chin is poorly developed, and the nasal opening is broad. The head is inclined to be narrow, the upper jaw protrudes, and the forehead is rounded. The arms are rather long and slender and the pelvis is narrow.[1] These features immediately differentiate the negroids from other groups of people, although there are people with some of these attributes in parts of tropical south-east Asia and in the Pacific region. The Sahara Desert forms a natural northern limit to their range. The pygmies of the Congo forests and the bushmen of south-west Africa are distinct from the negroids and are almost certainly of a separate evolutionary origin. Some anthropologists consider the diminutive pygmies and bushmen as ancestral to the larger negroids, but it is more likely that they are survivors of more abundant and widespread populations that have become reduced

[1] This is a short biological description of negroid features and must be interpreted as such.

and restricted in range through the activities of the larger negroids. This view is adopted by Cole (1963) upon whose discussion of the origin and diversity of the human population of Africa much of the following account is based.

Fossil *Homo sapiens* from the Kenya Rift Valley dated as Palaeolithic or Mesolithic are caucasoid and show no trace of the typical negroid features. The oldest known negroid skeleton was found near Timbuktu and is estimated to be early post-Pleistocene, that is to say it is relatively recent. This specimen differs in a number of features from the people that now live in the area, and the modern negroid is likely to have evolved much more recently. The almost complete absence of fossil evidence means that it is impossible to say when and where the negroids evolved, but all the evidence suggests that they have colonized Africa quite recently. Various attempts have been made to use blood group gene frequencies as a means of estimating their relationship with other peoples, but as will be shown in Chapter 10, blood group genes are susceptible to natural selection and therefore probably have the capacity for rapid evolutionary changes in frequency. The only possibility that exists that might help in tracing negroid origins would be the discovery of fossils in Africa or elsewhere that are undoubtedly negroid and which can be accurately dated.

The negroids are divided into a number of groups based partly on the structure of the language, partly on physical (including genetic) features, and partly on geographical distribution. A very much simplified map of the distribution of the main groups of people is shown in Fig. 4. The pygmies are omitted because they now occur only in scattered pockets in the Congo region. The West African group occupies an area from about the Senegal River across northern tropical Africa to the Nile. This group intergrades considerably with the Bantu group to the south, indeed the two have much in common as is reflected in similar sorts of wood carvings and in the persistence of complex secret societies. The West African group occurs particularly along the humid coast of West Africa. In the savanna to the north there has been much mixture with Muslims from the north, and the result is that the savanna people are on the whole more caucasoid. There are however numerous problems associated with attempts to define the West African group. Thus the Hausa of

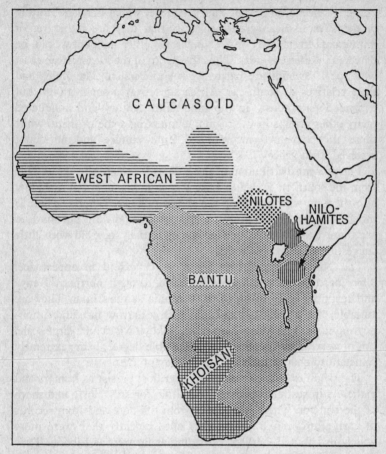

Fig. 4 Distribution map of the main groups of people in Africa.
(*Adapted from Cole, 1963.*)

Northern Nigeria speak a Hamitic language, but in terms of physical features they are West African negroids.

The Bantu are immensely variable and occupy an enormous range south of the West African group extending to the extreme south of south-east Africa where they are represented by the Zulus. In East Africa they are mixed with Hamites and it is possible that they are partly descended from the caucasoids that lived in the area in early post-Pleistocene times, but their language, which is related to that of the West African group, suggests that they are rather recent immigrants from the west. Numerous other influences can be detected in different areas. Thus the Bantu of the East African coast who speak Swahili are partly Arab and Persian. The Zulus and their relatives of south-east Africa started as a small group, but expanded enormously in the nineteenth century and conquered many other groups in the region, eliminating some of them, while those that remained incorporated Zulu culture and no doubt received Zulu genes.

The present distribution of the Nilotes is around the White Nile from the southern Sudan to Lake Kyoga in Uganda, but including also the Luo who live along the shores of Lake Victoria. There is much variation in this group; many are tall and thin, but the Luo are more heavily built, and all are essentially negroid with little suggestion of caucasoid traits.

The Nilo-Hamites are rather more caucasoid in appearance. They occur from south-eastern Sudan through northern Kenya and reappear again in northern Tanzania as the Masai. They are variable, but usually tall and thin with a narrow face and a non-negroid nose. The Masai have taken Kikuyu wives on a large scale, but preserve their identity to a remarkable degree, being extremely reluctant to change their traditional way of life.

The pygmies (sometimes called negrillos) persist as hunters and gatherers in scattered pockets in the rain forest 5° north and south of the equator. There is evidence from folk lore and from records of early European travellers that until recently they were more widely distributed, perhaps extending as far west as Liberia. They are remarkably well adjusted to the forest environment and although there has been some mixture with the surrounding Bantu-speaking cultivators they have managed to remain distinct, albeit in small numbers. Two distinctive types of pygmy can be recognized: one round-headed with narrow shoulders, short legs, and almost no beard or body hair, the other with a longer head, broad shoulders, more muscular and hairy, and rather paler-skinned. Both groups have a paler skin than that of the surrounding negroids and the eyes are rather bulging, a feature which perhaps is associated with the gloomy environment inside the forest. The original language of the pygmies has almost disappeared and they now speak languages that are derived from the surrounding Bantu-speakers.

The Khoisans consist of the bushmen and Hottentots who are placed together not only because of physical similarities but also because of the use of 'clicks' in their languages. There is evidence that the Khoisan people have been isolated in the southern part of Africa for a long time. Numerous rock paintings and evidence of the use of tools and weapons have been found that date them at least as far back as the middle or upper Pleistocene (Clark, 1960). There is also evidence that they occupied a much greater area than now, the bushmen in particular having been reduced in numbers and restricted to the deserts of south-western Africa by pressures from both the negroids and the Europeans.

Summarizing, it would appear that the negroids, the people that are generally thought of as Africans, have appeared on the scene relatively recently. They possibly evolved in the forest region of West Africa sometime during the late Pleistocene and thence spread over most of the continent in recent times, but failed to cross the Sahara to North Africa. The two main groups, the West African and the Bantu-speakers, have much in common, but within each there is physical and cultural diversity. The present small size of populations of pygmies and bushmen is probably the result of the invasion of their areas by the negroids. In the south there has been considerable mixing of negroid and Khoisan genes, but nothing like the same amount of mixing has occurred with the pygmies. There has obviously been repeated infiltration of North African and western Asiatic caucasoids across the Sahara. This infiltration is reflected not only in the genetic make-up of the numerous and diverse populations, but also in religious beliefs, culture, and in the ways in which the environment is utilized.

Tropical Africa is also thinly populated with Europeans and Asians. The Europeans were until recently administrators, representatives of commercial enterprises, missionaries, and settlers. Many of these still remain, but there are also teachers and advisers. The extent to which they have integrated both culturally and genetically varies from place to place. The Portuguese have perhaps integrated most successfully as can be seen in the streets of Lisbon where many of the people show traces of negroid features. On the whole the genetic impact of the European colonization and exploitation of Africa has been small, but the economic effects have been enormous. The Europeans brought with them literacy, Christianity, and the basic notion that the environment should be exploited, and they are largely responsible for the present ecological predicament that faces tropical Africa. Their most important ecological achievement is that they have reduced the death rate among the negroid populations with the result that the population which for generations had been maintained at relative stability suddenly expanded and created numerous problems, most of which had not been anticipated. West (1965) refers to the Europeans as the 'white tribes' of Africa. His delightfully written book provides a considerable insight into their varied activities in the new nations of Africa.

There are also large numbers of Asians who are mainly involved in commercial activities. The Indians in East Africa have for long had almost complete control of the retail business and their present unpopularity among the negroids is partly because they failed to integrate into the new nations created at independence. They have remained genetically distinct from the negroids and have kept up their customs and beliefs. Their future seems uncertain. All along the West African coast the Lebanese have occupied a similar niche. Many families are third or fourth generation, and many have never seen and have no prospect of seeing their land of origin. Some are extremely rich, but they are careful not to allow too much money to accumulate in West Africa, and their custom is to have bank accounts overseas. The Asian immigrants and their descendants have high birth rates and considerably lower death rates than the negroids, mainly because they have more money to spend on food and medicine.

Almost all the nations of tropical Africa were until recently colonies that were administered by European powers, notably Britain, France, and Belgium. The Portuguese, despite much international opposition, still maintain territories in Mozambique, Angola, and Guinea. The European colonial powers divided the continent up after a series of disputes and political agreements, and in so doing took little notice of the ethnic differences of the people within their territories. The result is that the territorial limits of the present independent nations of Africa (Fig. 1) are to a large extent arbitrary, many national boundaries cutting right through populations of the same ethnic group, and at the same time including within them people that are more different from each other than, for instance, the English and the Russians. The differences between these groups not only involve language, but also religious beliefs and modes of life.

The political instability that is a feature of the modern African nations is partly generated by internal disputes that arise because the people within the nation are so different from each other. This situation is not of course peculiar to Africa: it occurs everywhere to some extent, but because people are more readily identifiable as belonging to a particular ethnic group in Africa than in many other areas of the world, its effects are more conspicuous. Thus the Ibos and the Hausas were simply unable to come to terms with each other, a situation which was partly responsible for a civil war and much loss of life. The Hausas are mainly Muslims and derive much of their culture from the Arabs while the Ibos have to a large extent accepted the Christian faith or have retained their polytheism. The attitudes to life of the two groups are totally different: thus the Hausas are polygamous and by most standards the women are treated badly, while the Ibo women are remarkably independent and are frequently more opportunist than the men in business matters. Ibo women work harder than the men while Hausa wives often regard it as a privilege to be exempt from heavy work. Ethnic conflicts have assumed considerable proportions in the Sudan where the Muslims are trying hard to dominate the Christians and polytheists of the south, a situation which has resulted in an enormous flow of refugees over the border from the Sudan into Uganda where problems of feeding and providing shelter have arisen. This pattern of ethnic conflict repeats itself throughout tropical Africa and is doubtless a serious hindrance to economic development and political stability.

The new African nations started with European concepts of democratic government, but after repeated disputes these have in many places been replaced by military dictatorships and one-party systems of government. There is now unfortunately much political corruption and elections are often fought on an ethnic basis rather than on differences in political policy. The army has often intervened and taken control, and although this does away with the necessity for elections and politicians, it tends to create rivalries for power within the army which lead to coups and counter-coups. Some politicians urge an end to what they call tribalism but it seems that ethnic differences will remain and will continue to play a part in the economic and political future of Africa. Other leaders have advocated the retention of tribal and ethnic groups on the grounds that these promote social welfare.

In addition, conflicts between the more settled cultivators and the nomadic pastoralists are likely to continue as the population's of both grow. The pastoralists live chiefly in the savanna region, much of which is not suitable for cultivation because of an inadequate water supply, but as the numbers of the cultivators increase they become more and more expansionist and are extending their sphere of activities into areas that for long have been occupied by the pastoralists. It is not easy to imagine the two ecologically different groups coming to terms: their interests are totally different, and they are to a large extent of separate ethnic origin. But perhaps more importantly there will arise conflicts between the wealthy élite (which includes politicians, government officials, business men, and others) and the peasant majority. There are few areas in the world where the gap between the few rich and the many poor is as wide as it is in tropical Africa.

The United Nations designates all the countries of Africa as 'developing', but it makes an exception of South Africa which is regarded as a 'developed' country. It is not clear exactly what is meant by a developing country, but in terms of economics the word is synonymous with under-developed. Economic development is often thought of as a cumulative process that increases individual consumption, but it is quite clear that if all the people in the world were to suddenly start consuming the resources of the world at the rate they are being consumed in North America and Europe these resources would quickly be used up. Developed nations thus depend upon the existence of under-developed nations for their resources of raw materials and if certain countries are to remain developed in the sense understood by the economists it becomes imperative that most people in the world must not use the world's resources at anything like the same rate. It has been pointed out for instance that if the Chinese used oil at the same rate as the Americans the world's supply of oil would be exhausted in a few years.

The income per head of the population is frequently used as a measure of which countries are developed and which under-developed. Developed countries are defined as those with an income per head of over a thousand U.S. dollars a year. In most under-developed countries income is below 200 dollars a year. Incomes per head (in 1962) for most of the tropical African countries are shown in Table 2. As pointed out by Hodder (1968) the figures provide only a rough estimate of development or of under-development as they show only one aspect of the standard of living: the average amount of money available to an individual in a year. The majority of the people of tropical Africa provide their own food and many have no money in an average year and yet are able to feed themselves and their families. And then there are people in all of these countries with very large incomes. These include politicians, administrators, doctors, some teachers, and an unknown number engaged in commercial enterprises of various sorts. But despite these considerations the income per head can be used as a measure of the ability of the individual to buy and consume materials produced elsewhere, and this, according to the economists, is one way of assessing development. Compared with tropical America the average incomes in tropical Africa are low and are paralleled only by a few countries in south-east Asia. In 1962 Ghana stood out as having the highest incomes; this was probably because under the Nkrumah régime an attempt was made to develop minor industries to provide jobs.

More recent (1966) figures issued by the International Bank for Reconstruction and Development and expressed in terms of 'per capita gross national product' suggest that the values (in dollars) are considerably higher than those shown in Table 2, but relative to the world trend there has been little change. Within tropical Africa it is doubtful if Ghana still maintains its lead, and in all probability the people of many African countries have relatively lower average incomes (at the time of writing) than they did ten years ago. But figures of this sort must not be taken too seriously as apart from difficulties in knowing exactly what they mean to the average person in a country, there must be considerable difficulty in arriving at a figure in the first place, especially when one bears in mind uncertainties over population census results.

Another concept of a developing or under-developed country is that it has the potential for economic development, even though this potential is often elusive. Hodder (1968) defines under-development in both economic and biological terms and this, it seems to me, is closer to the truth. He suggests that people in under-developed countries have a low life expectancy at birth, poor health, and that they are largely illiterate. Their food is obtained mainly by subsistence agriculture and the economy is not diversified, but is geared to the production of a small range of raw materials. There is little or no industry and no large-scale application of modern technology to agriculture and industry. To this I would add that the rate of population growth is higher than the world average and that there is little or no attempt to limit this growth. Estimated annual rates of population increase for tropical African countries are given in Table 1, but as will be discussed in Chapter 2, these estimates are likely to be unreliable, and probably too low. The population of tropical Africa is rapidly getting to a level where subsistence production of food and the export of raw materials for consumption by developed countries cannot continue as they are if the present low standards of living are to be maintained, let alone improved.

The most pervasive aspect of life in modern Africa is perhaps the economic role that the different countries are forced to play. Tropical Africa earns foreign currency from developed countries by selling its natural resources in the form of raw materials, chiefly plant products, but also minerals and oil. The economy of many African countries is largely dependent upon the export of a single natural resource, the world market for which may fluctuate unpredictably. In the case of plant products there is the continual danger of devastation of the crop by pests and diseases which also leads to uncertainty for the future. From an ecological point of view most tropical African countries can be designated as producers of materials that are consumed by the developed countries, and, as will be discussed in the final chapter of this book, this is creating an un-precedented dilemma now that the human population is rapidly increasing. As the industrial markets of the developed countries become more and more consolidated there will be increasing pressure on the under-developed countries to produce more and more raw materials. But this is unlikely to result in a general rise in the standard of living in the under-developed countries as it will become increasingly difficult for them to begin to compete in the industrial and business arena which is already so highly organized. It would therefore seem that the present trend in world business will keep the under-developed countries of Africa and elsewhere in the role of producers of raw materials and that the already-rich in the developed countries will become even richer. How long this state of affairs will persist is a matter for speculation but what is certain is that today's business conspiracy in the developed countries is not concerned with the long-term effects of its activity of utilizing the world's resources as quickly as possible.

The relationship between human ecology and economic development is discussed more fully in the last chapter of this book. Here it is simply necessary to indicate that prospects for economic development in tropical Africa must be considered in relation to the African environment and the people that live in this environment. The following nine chapters explore aspects of the ecology of the tropical African environment.

CHAPTER 2

Population

Most populations of plants and animals have an enormous capacity for increasing in size which, however, is rarely realized: the world is not full of mango trees and locusts. This is because populations are for the most part regulated in size in such a way that a tendency to increase in numbers usually results in an increase in the death rate, and the long-term result is an equilibrium which is adjusted to the available resources, especially to the food supply.

Man belongs to a single species in which all members can potentially interbreed. Geographical and cultural barriers tend to inhibit interbreeding, although these barriers are being progressively broken down. Man therefore consists of a single population, broken into smaller populations which are to a considerable extent isolated from each other. No other animal of comparable size is as abundant as man. It is possible to single out the development of agriculture, the invention of medicines, and the utilization of energy other than through eating as the three most important ecological events that have allowed the enormous recent expansion in human numbers. Modern man also differs from most other organisms in that he tends to modify his environment to suit himself rather than to fit into the existing environment. The extent of man's modification of the environment differs in various parts of the world, but almost everywhere the impact of man on the natural ecosystem can be seen. Extreme examples of this modification are the big cities in which almost all living things except man have been destroyed, and also cultivated areas where natural vegetation and its associated animals have been removed and replaced by crops and the pests and weeds of crops. The recent increase in the abundance of man is thus the most important biological event since the origin of life.

In 1965 the world population was estimated at 3285 million and by 1980 it should be well over 4000 million. In 1964 the overall birth rate was about 34 per thousand and the death rate about 16 per thousand. This means that in 1964 the world population was increasing at a rate of 1·8 per cent per year. All the evidence suggests that the rate of increase is itself increasing. In 1968 about 70 million people were added to the world population, and using this figure it would appear that the population will double in 36 years if not before. The most important population parameter for most countries is the rate of increase. The rate is by no means constant throughout the world, being on the whole higher in the poorer and lower in the richer countries. In many poor countries the rate of increase is around 3 per cent per year and the expected doubling time of the population is correspondingly decreased. The rapid increase in human numbers is not being caused by an increase in the birth rate but by a spectacular decrease in the death rate, especially the death rate of children. Many more individuals survive to reproduce than a hundred years ago and the number surviving and reproducing is increasing every year.

In the past twenty years numerous books have been published that draw attention to the disastrous situation that is developing as human numbers continue to rise. Famine is expected to be widespread by the end of the present decade and it has become increasingly apparent that the dependence of many countries on gifts of food supplies from other countries will have to end in the near future. North America has for years been responsible for keeping countless numbers of people alive in India and other over-populated and poor countries by sending large quantities of surplus food, but it is felt that soon all the food produced by North America will be required to feed the ever-increasing numbers of North Americans. Improving food production is often cited as a means of overcoming the problem, but it is obvious that since an improvement in food production will simply lead to better survival, its effects can at best be judged as short-term. Assuming that no one really wants to increase the death rate, especially the death rate of children, the only possible approach is to decrease the birth rate. This could in theory solve the problem, at least in limited areas, but probably not on a world basis because most people in the world do not have the knowledge to even appreciate the problem and certainly not the money or inclination to practise birth control. In addition there are people, including some economists, but especially influential theologians, who oppose birth control. Economists are apt to suggest that education and economic development should proceed as rapidly as possible so as to keep up with rising human numbers, while theologians are apt to argue that birth control is against the will of God.

Almost all religions, including those that in Africa the Christians and the Muslims regard as pagan, encourage the production of as many children as possible, and it is sometimes supposed that this is an adaptation (by implication an evolutionary adaptation) to the expected high death rates. But although in man this may be so to some extent the evidence from other animals suggests that the birth rates are adjusted independently by natural selection and are not determined by the expected death rates. This may also be so in man as the decrease in the death rate that has occurred throughout the world in the last few generations has in most cases not been compensated for by a fall in the birth rate, except in a few areas where birth control has become acceptable. The possibilities for a large-scale programme of birth control in tropical Africa seem remote; indeed the Regional Director for Africa of the World Health Organization in an essay on Africa and the problem of contraception starts by being apologetic for raising what he calls an 'allegedly taboo subject' (Quenum, 1967).

Tropical Africa is not as densely populated as many areas of the world, but the rate of population increase is high by world standards. There is much regional variation in the density of people in different parts of Africa. Such variations in dispersion can be generally interpreted as the result of differences in the availability of food and risk of killing diseases. The ecological changes that have occurred in tropical Africa since the introduction of carbohydrate staple food crops have undoubtedly caused concentrations of people in areas where these can be grown most effectively. Disease contributes to variations in population density as large populations would be unable to become established in areas where most individuals die before reproducing themselves. These generalizations derive from the kind of situation frequently encountered in other animals. But nowadays the situation is less clear because the effects of disease are no longer as marked as they must have been in the past, and, moreover, food can be transported from place to place.

1 Victims of the Nigerian civil war. These people had fled into the bush and when they reappeared they were on the verge of starvation.

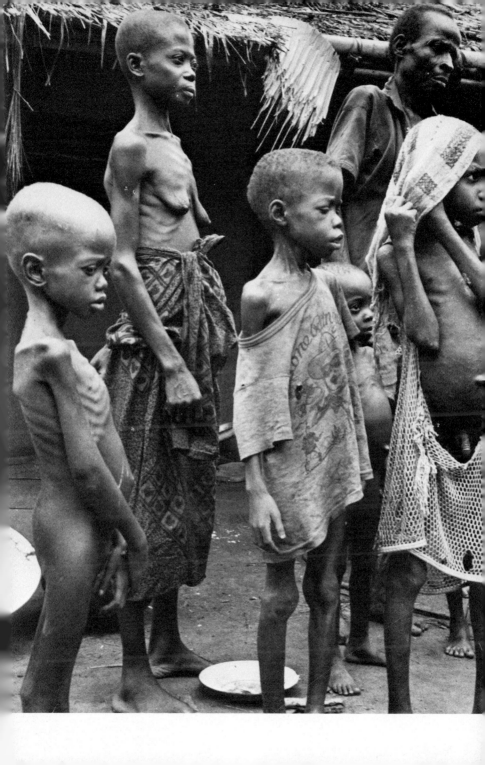

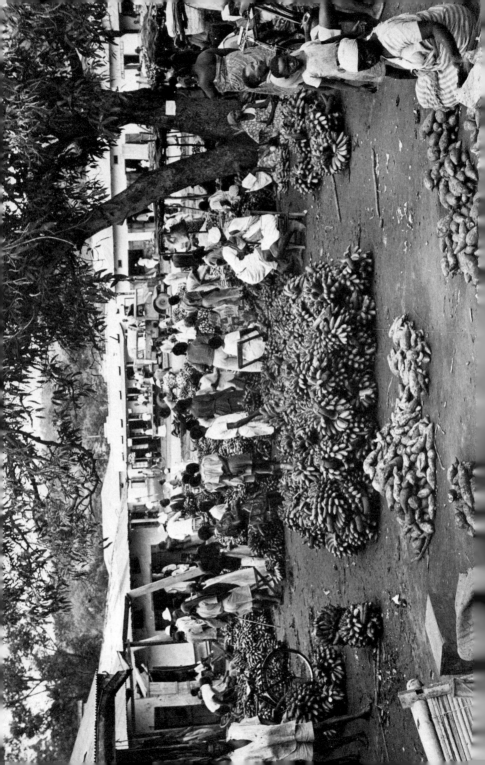

There is no area in the world in which vital information on human numbers is so sparse as in tropical Africa. Even the estimates of the number of people in some countries are probably highly inaccurate, and information on birth and death rates is probably unreliable (Brass *et al.*, 1968). Except in certain limited areas that have been especially studied there is little information on such parameters as the cause of death, the age at death, and life expectancy. A Demographic Yearbook showing world population trends is published periodically by the United Nations and it is clear from this that vital information about the population of tropical Africa is scanty. There are numerous difficulties: most people live in rural and remote areas and this makes the gathering of information during a census difficult, many people, including some administrators, local chiefs, and elders, being reluctant to give information because they do not understand why the information is necessary and in any case distrust people who ask what they regard as personal questions. Most rural people are illiterate and many do not know their own age or the ages of their children. In addition some censuses until recently recorded information only about the European population and ignored the indigenous people. Much effort is now being devoted to improving census techniques in Africa.

Table 1 shows the estimated population and population density in each of the thirty-four countries of tropical Africa. Some of these countries, notably Sudan, Mali, Upper Volta, Niger, Chad, and the Somali Republic, have large areas of uninhabitable desert and the population is concentrated around rivers and lakes or the coast. As shown there is much variation in population density between the countries. Rwanda, the second smallest country of tropical Africa, has the highest density of people, but of the larger countries, Nigeria has the biggest population and the highest density. The annual rates of population increase are also shown in Table 1. In most countries the rate seems to be just over 2 per cent per year, but rates of over 3 per cent per year have been calculated for the Ivory Coast, Niger, Rhodesia, Rwanda, and the Somali Republic. The very low rate of 0·2 per cent per year for Portuguese Guinea is probably wrong, but it may be noted that low rates are also recorded for Angola and Mozambique, the other two Portuguese territories in Africa. Indeed the reliability of all of these rates is open to

2 A market scene in tropical Africa. Cassava, bananas, and sweet potatoes are stacked everywhere. There is plenty of food, but the food contains little protein.

considerable doubt: why for instance should the Ivory Coast have an annual rate of increase of 3·3 per cent while its neighbour, Liberia, has a rate of only 1·4 per cent? The answer in this case is that Liberia has never had an adequate census of its population.

Table 3 shows the estimated birth and death rates and the expectation of further life for the people of 23 tropical African countries for which such information is available. These figures are based on samples of various sizes of varying degrees of reliability and were obtained over a period of about ten years between 1955 and 1965. At best the figures are between five and fifteen years out of date, but more importantly it is likely that they are based largely on the situation in or near large towns where some attempt at registering births and deaths is made. What happens in the rural areas is anyone's guess, but one can be sure that death rates are higher than those shown in Table 3. The birth rates in all the countries shown are higher than the world average of 34 per thousand and almost all the death rates are higher than the world average of 16 per thousand. The birth rates vary between countries far less than the death rates: indeed the birth rates probably approximate the maximum possible production in human populations. Variations in the death rate between countries are largely determined by the ecological conditions in these countries. Table 3 also shows the infant death rates, which in most countries are very high, reaching about a quarter of all children born in some cases, and the expectation of life at birth, which is conspicuously low, especially in males. As will be shown in Chapter 3, the infant mortality can be much higher than is indicated in Table 3, especially in remote rural areas.

There are rarely uncertainties about the sex of an individual and the United Nations Demographic Yearbooks provide information on sex ratios for most African countries. There are some variations from country to country but in general the ratio seems close to the expected 1:1. The survival of the two sexes at different ages varies markedly, but reliable information on the age structure of the population is less easy to assemble. Variations in the sex ratio in relation to age in Sierra Leone are discussed later in this chapter.

In man there is a slight but statistically significant excess of males over the expected 1:1 ratio at birth. Taking the world population as a whole 51·46 per cent of births are males, but there is evidence that the sex ratio of zygotes is much higher and that there is in fact a selective mortality of male embryos before birth. Numerous factors have been suggested to explain local variations and variations with age in the sex ratio, some of them genetic and others environmental. Fisher (1930) explained that no matter what the mechanism of sex determination, an approximately 1:1 ratio of the sexes would be maintained by natural selection. The almost universal occurrence of 1:1 ratios tends to be taken for granted, but Fisher's explanation, which is widely accepted, becomes relevant when deviations from the expected are encountered. His reasoning is as follows:

Suppose male births are less frequent than female. A newborn male then has better mating prospects than a female and can expect to have more offspring. Any parent producing more males would tend to have more grandchildren. Since sex is inherited the male-producing tendencies spread and male births become more frequent in the population. As the 1:1 ratio is approached the initial advantage of the males is reduced. The same reasoning of course applies if we start with a deficiency of females. Therefore the sex ratio is maintained by selection at the 1:1 equilibrium.

The main ecological effect of the introduction of Christianity into Africa has been that since this religion demands that each man shall have only one wife there has been an increase in monogamous marriages. But the impact of Christianity must not be exaggerated; indeed the evolution of a monogamous society has probably more to do with rising affluence in the towns than to religion. People living in the towns are tending more and more to substitute material things for large families, and polygamy is becoming less frequent in urban areas. Large areas of tropical Africa are populated by Muslims whose religion permits polygamy, as indeed do many of the so-called pagan religions. Polygamy should mean that many men remain unmarried, and this may be so, but in all probability most men are responsible for some children.

Most men marry within their own community and usually within their own ethnic group. This helps to maintain the identity and cultural distinctiveness of the group. People living in towns or those exposed to outside cultures are the only ones to marry relatively often outside their own group. Even university students will frequently announce that they are going back to their village to find a wife.

Most girls marry when very young, often at puberty, while men marry at about thirty because they have to accumulate bride-wealth. In many parts of Africa the first child is born early during a woman's reproductive life and she continues to have children until she is physiologically unable to do so. The total number of children born to a woman therefore depends to a large extent on the spacing of successive births. There is considerable circumstantial evidence for deliberate spacing of children, especially among women in rural areas where there is a high infant mortality rate. In particular it is the custom in many areas for a woman not to become pregnant again until her last child has been completely weaned. This custom has presumably evolved as a result of high death rates among children whose mothers become pregnant while they are still lactating. On the other hand if a child is stillborn or if it dies within about a year of birth (while still being breast-fed) the mother soon becomes pregnant again. Births are thus deliberately spaced but if the youngest child dies it is immediately replaced.

The intervals between successive births have been recorded in the Western Nigerian village of Imesi (Martin, Morley, and Woodland, 1964). The information obtained is reproduced in Tables 4 and 5. As shown in Table 4 the interval before the birth of another baby is much shorter if the first baby dies or is stillborn, the mean interval before the next birth being less than half the interval between surviving children. But even when the child survives there is evidence from this sample that the interval, on average six months more, is longer than in a comparable population from Cocos-Keeling in the South Pacific. This suggests that there is a deliberate spacing of children which reduces the total number of children born but increases the probability of survival to maturity. At Imesi the mean duration of lactation is nearly two years, which appears to be longer than in most human societies. But the importance of a long lactation period is considerable in an area where alternative methods of feeding babies are not readily available. The few women that do become pregnant during lactation meet a certain amount of public censure and may even have to leave the village.

Most human births are of single individuals, but twins are relatively frequent, and triplets and higher numbers up to five or six also occur rarely. There is evidence that multiple births are more frequent among West African women than elsewhere in the world, particularly among the Yoruba of Western Nigeria. The published frequencies of multiple births are usually based on hospital admissions which are likely to be biased as women about to produce more than one child are more likely to seek admission to hospital. Since the survival of African babies is in general hazardous the apparent high frequency of twinning is of special interest.

Hollingsworth and Duncan (1966) record seven sets of triplets, 291 pairs of twins and 5256 single births at a maternity hospital at Accra in Ghana during 1954–6. This gives a multiple pregnancy rate of 1 in 18·6, which is high, and possibly reflects this tendency to seek hospital care if a multiple birth is expected. It was estimated that 28·7 per cent of the twins were monozygotic and compared with other samples (all European) there was a statistically significant low frequency of female–female twins which could not be explained. The mortality rate of these twins was about 15 per cent which is similar to that found in samples from Italy, but lower than the 21 per cent found in English twins. Hollingsworth and Duncan suggest that the rather high rate of survival of the Ghanaian twins is because they are not conspicuously underweight and that twinning is more 'natural' in Ghanaian than in European women.

Knox and Morley (1960) record the frequency of twinning among babies born to Yoruba women at Ilesha, Western Nigeria. The frequency of twinning rose markedly with birth rank from 2·4 per cent of first pregnancies to just over 11 per cent among mothers who already had seven or more children. A slight increase in the probability of twinning with birth rank has been found in England and elsewhere, but the rise is nothing like as steep as in Yoruba women. Knox and Morley also found a seasonal cycle in the probability of twinning, as shown in Table 6. Twins are statistically more frequent in the period May to October than during the remainder of the year. It is tempting to ascribe this seasonal variation to variations in rainfall and temperature which in turn affect disease transmission and nutrition in the community, but correlations of this sort are difficult to interpret, and in the absence of evidence the cause of the seasonal variation cannot be identified. The high incidence of twinning among the Yoruba women has often been commented upon and recently it has been confirmed (Nylander, 1971) that the high rate compared with other areas of Nigeria is due to an increase in the frequency of dizygotic twins, the rates for monozygotic twins being more or less constant throughout the country.

In some areas twins are considered undesirable or unlucky and there is a considerable body of largely anecdotal evidence that they are killed off. In parts of Nigeria missionaries have in the past devoted much effort to persuade people not to kill twins. The extent to which twin-killing occurred or still occurs is not known, but such behaviour might, through the process of natural selection, reduce the frequency of twinning as there is a hereditary component to the likelihood of twins.

I now wish to discuss the population of a single country, drawing particular attention to the difficulties encountered when attempts are made to obtain a clear picture of the situation. The country I have chosen, Sierra Leone, is representative of what is prevalent throughout tropical Africa, although of course there are numerous differences between countries.

Sierra Leone lies mainly within the forest region of West Africa, but most of the forest has been cut down and the land cultivated, although often abandoned again as the soil becomes unproductive. Most of the people are cultivators and subsistence farming is the main occupation. Some crop products are exported, but the bulk of Sierra Leone's small revenue comes from the export of minerals, especially of diamonds. There is a heavy concentration of people in and around the capital city, Freetown, which was first settled at the end of the eighteenth century by people of varied ethnic origin, many of them freed slaves, and a large proportion originating from Nigeria. These people, the creoles, dominate the commercial and administrative life of the country, but their numbers are relatively small and there is evidence of a decline in their former influence. Their position can be understood in the context of the special relationship that developed between them and the British colonial administrators who in effect deliberately turned them into an élite ruling class.

The origin of the bulk of the population of Sierra Leone is obscure. It is believed that the country has been subjected to repeated waves of immigration from the north, east, and south-east, and that the people that remained evolved into ethnic (tribal) groups with distinctive languages and customs. The groups maintained their differences through fear and suspicion of one another, sometimes by war, and frequently by co-operation within the group. The two most numerous groups, the Temne and the Mende, occupied the west-central and southern regions, respectively, and although with the opening up of the country by road and rail there has been much movement in recent years, the strong geographical component to the distribution of these two groups remains. Some ethnic groups have become more dispersed than others: the Kono are still concentrated into a rather small area in the east, but the Fula, who are inclined to become traders, are well dispersed over the whole country, although they are still most numerous in the north. With the introduction of parliamentary democracy, political parties became strongly associated with ethnic groups and this has caused difficulties at elections, as for instance in 1967 when the Temne voted for one party and the Mende for the other. Indeed the 1967 elections perhaps provide support for the notion that the existence of several political parties within a country encourages tribalism and this may help to explain why so many African countries have abandoned the multi-party in favour of the one-party system. The distinctiveness of the ethnic groups is however chiefly maintained by language differences, and even in Freetown, where all the ethnic groups are represented, each tends to remain discrete and loyal, associating and marrying within the group to an astonishing degree.

The first census of the population of Sierra Leone was held in 1963. Earlier sample censuses suggested that the population should be about 2·5 million, and when it was announced that the census revealed a population of only 2 180 355 there was much criticism of its accuracy. Some politicians felt that the low numbers recorded would lower the prestige of Sierra Leone and reduce possibilities of external investment and aid. The figure obtained is likely to be on the low side because a large number of people live in remote areas, and since they are mainly illiterate they tended to be suspicious of census enumerators, who in some cases were rather inexperienced.

The most serious discrepancy between the estimated figures and the actual census results occurred in the predominantly Mende southern province of the country. In 1960 it was estimated that there were nearly 850 thousand people in this province, but the 1963 census revealed the presence of a little less than 550 thousand people. Only in Freetown were the 1963 figures markedly higher than those estimated in 1960. No information was obtained on birth and death rates, but a rough estimate suggested that the population was expanding at a rate of about 2 per cent per year, which, if true, should produce a population of about three million by 1980. As would be expected the highest density of people is in Freetown; elsewhere high densities occur north-east of Freetown where rice, fish, palm kernels, and iron are important products, and in the diamond areas of the east.

The ethnic composition of the population of Sierra Leone is shown in Table 7. These figures are based largely on the language spoken by each person and on what he claimed to be. Nevertheless they are probably reasonably accurate. As shown in Table 7 only 1·3 per cent of the population could not be classified into an ethnic group. These and the 'others' are probably mainly Lebanese who have settled in Freetown and other centres of business as traders and dealers, and Europeans and Indians who live mainly in Freetown. The creoles, who play such a paramount part in the running of the nation, comprise only 1·9 per cent of the total. But what is most remarkable is that almost everyone in the country can be classified either by language or by their own admission into an identifiable ethnic group.

It is frequently announced in Sierra Leone that someone has died at a very advanced age indeed. Judged from these announcements considerable numbers of people live to over a hundred years and some to 120 or more. Almost certainly these ages are exaggerated. Old age is often associated with authority and wisdom and once past the age of about sixty many people are proud to be old and are apt to pretend that they are much older. Declarations of age during the 1963 census were treated with caution. Illiteracy and inadequate registration facilities in the rural areas result in many people not knowing their real age and this, added to the tendency to exaggerate, gave the census enumerators problems when attempting to assess age. The problem was partly overcome by asking people if they were born before or after certain local events, but the high frequency of ages declared in fives and tens suggests that many guesses were necessary. The results of the 1963 census as regards the age structure of the entire population are shown in Table 8. As pointed out by Clarke (1966) the most striking feature of the age structure of the population is the high proportion of young people. Thus in 1963, 36·7 per cent of the people were under 15, 54·3 per cent under 25, and 71·7 per cent under 35. This contrasts with a country like Britain where the comparable figures are 23·0 per cent, 37·2 per cent, and 49·7 per cent. Apart from the very old, whose ages are likely to be exaggerated, there are fewer older people in Sierra Leone than in Britain, only 7·7 per cent being 60 years or more compared with 17·6 per cent in Britain. All the available evidence is suggestive of a high birth rate and a high death rate, but it is only in the Freetown area that figures are available. Here (using only registered births and deaths) the birth rate was 41·4 per thousand in 1962 and the death rate 18·6 per thousand. But hospital and medical facilities are better in Freetown than elsewhere in the country and the death rate may be correspondingly lower. But even in Freetown, 115 infants in every thousand die before they are one year old, and there is no doubt that in rural areas the death rate of infants is much higher. Within Sierra Leone there is considerable geographical variation in the age structure of the population which can be accounted for partly by the movements of young males in search of work, particularly by movements into the diamond areas and into Freetown.

The 1963 census revealed an excess of 18 109 females which gives an overall sex ratio of 1017 females to 1000 males. The excess of females is much lower than in Europe where the expectation of life of women is longer than that of men. Geographical variation in the sex ratio within Sierra Leone is mainly correlated with the migration of males into Freetown and into other centres that offer work and opportunities. If one accepts the age distribution revealed by the census it is then possible to separate the age groups by sex, as shown in Table 9. It can be assumed that the slight excess of males at birth known to occur in man also occurs in the Sierra Leone population, but as shown in Table 9 the assumed preponderance of male births quickly disappears and for the first five years of life there is an excess of females. Then from the age of 5 to 14 there is a considerable excess of males followed by an excess of females between the ages of 15 and 34. From 35 onwards males greatly outnumber females, especially in the 45–59 age group, and in old age there is a slight increase in the relative frequency of females, but they remain less frequent than males. Clarke (1966) attempts to interpret these changes, and cautions that in the case of females in the 15–34 age group there are likely to be inaccuracies in the estimates of age, especially by young married women, and also that at the time the census was taken the activities of the Bundu Society (female initiation society) may have affected the results. But the preponderance of males from 35 onwards is so marked that a biological effect is suggested. The most likely cause of the excess of males from 35 onwards is an increased probability of death among the older women as a result of excessive child bearing and heavy manual labour among those in the rural areas. By the age of 35 almost all the women will have given birth to a considerable number of children and any further pregnancies are probably a serious threat to health.

CHAPTER 3

Life and Death in Rural Africa

Most people in tropical Africa live in rural surroundings. There has in recent years been a drift towards the towns in search of jobs, but in general the population is well dispersed. There seem to be people everywhere, and if one stops in an apparently remote and deserted area men, women, and children are likely to appear within a very short time.

These people live in villages of varying size, and most individuals do not have the chance to move far from the village where they were born. They support themselves in a variety of ways, depending on the area, and day-to-day existence does not depend on the transfer of money from one individual to another. They are in every sense 'under-developed', and for most of the time their existence is ignored by the more affluent minority in the towns and cities. The rural people have few medical facilities, little prospect of a reasonable education, and are usually in very poor health. They have an average income well below the low national average, and many adults rarely handle money. Their expectation of life is low, and the infant mortality rate may be as high as 40 per cent. The very high infant mortality rate in tropical Africa was in the past the main reason for the apparent stability of the human population size. The rapid growth of human numbers in recent years can be attributed partly to improved infant survival brought about by the introduction of drugs that suppress the effects of disease.

It is difficult to obtain information on life and death in rural Africa. In general, it is not possible to study a human population using the methods of the population ecologist investigating a natural population of an animal or a plant. Thus no doctor, biologist, or sociologist can impartially investigate mortality and the causes of mortality in a human society without at some point intervening and preventing individuals from dying. Hence such studies that have been made and the results that have been obtained will not represent exactly what is happening, but at the same time they provide the only information on the patterns of life and death in African villages. Doctors and sociologists have from time to time combined in long-term[1] studies of a village or community. These have revealed important interactions between disease, nutrition, social attitudes, and religious beliefs. They have also shown that the probability of death varies seasonally; indeed, in some areas the alternation of wet and dry seasons is the most significant ecological event affecting the people. There is almost everywhere a reluctance to report to European-trained doctors diseases believed to be caused by witchcraft or by administered 'punishment', and many rural people believe that such diseases cannot be cured by European methods.

The interaction of biological and social factors in human ecology is less apparent in analyses of human populations obtained by taking a much larger sample over a short period of time. Thus it is possible to determine the percentage of people in an area suffering from malaria or malnutrition, but this percentage must be treated with caution because it ignores seasonal effects. Indeed, sampling from a large population over a short period gives really reliable information on only the genetic traits present.

But the overriding problem is simply lack of information. Even routine information on the occurrence and spread of a disease is rarely collected and documented, and unfortunately there has in recent years been a marked tendency to withhold information on mortality resulting from disease. This information may be withheld by the people themselves because of the belief that the ills befalling them are the will of God and perhaps can only be cured by placating the gods, or by administrators who believe that the announcement of the presence of a dangerous disease may impede economic development by discouraging outside investment. Thomson (1967) cites a report of an outbreak of an unknown disease in a remote area south of the Niger near the Dahomey border. The report demonstrates one of the difficulties in obtaining sufficient information in time to identify and then to prevent the spread of the disease:

[1] Sometimes called 'longitudinal' studies by the medical profession, as opposed to 'cross-sectional' studies, which consist of sampling over a limited period.

Confirmation was obtained of the lethal effect of the epidemic which swept the banks of the Niger in October and November. . . . Many compounds were visited in which were freshly dug graves. In one compound there were eleven graves and one survivor. In the local lock-up both the jailer and his prisoner were buried within. Approximately 120 persons died in the neighbourhood of Illo itself and about 438 in the whole District. From reports from other areas it appears that at least 1,000 people must have died altogether. It appears to have been an epidemic form of pneumonia, and no medical officers were informed until the outbreak was almost over.

In the discussion following Thomson's paper (which was delivered at the Royal Society of Tropical Medicine and Hygiene) A. J. Duggan mentioned a similar event at Jos in Northern Nigeria. An outbreak of typhus in the township was discovered only after the inhabitants had run short of burial space and needed a new cemetery.

The spread of cholera into tropical Africa in 1970 is another example of the failure to reveal the true state of affairs. When cholera reached Sierra Leone there was at first no official statement and no news of mortality. The government, however, provided facilities for inoculation and encouraged people to make use of these by advertising on the radio. Unconfirmed reports suggested a high death rate in some parts of the country, but since there was no official information, rumours spread and the impact of the disease was probably much exaggerated. Later a few reports of deaths from cholera in Freetown were admitted, but no information ever appeared as to the status of the disease in rural areas.

In 1949 the Medical Research Council Laboratory at Fajara in The Gambia started investigations into many aspects of health and disease in a series of rural villages, some of which are relatively isolated. Additional villages have since been studied and a much clearer picture is now available about life in these villages than for any comparable area in tropical Africa. Although the investigations have been primarily medical it was realized that medical problems could not be considered in isolation, and so from time to time sociologists and others have joined the team. The results have been published in a series of papers which provide fundamental information on the ecology of rural populations and on the relationship between human ecology and sociology. Two general phenomena have emerged from these studies: the importance of seasonal changes in climate in the lives of the people, and the attitude of the villagers to health and disease which is totally different from that of Europeans. The account that follows is based largely on the work of the Medical Research Council Laboratory at Fajara, and particularly on the following papers: McGregor, Rahman *et al.* (1968), McGregor, Williams *et al.* (1966), Marsden (1964), Thompson (1966), Thompson and Rahman (1967), Thomson *et al.* (1968).

The village of Keneba is about 160 km from Bathurst, the capital of The Gambia. Its main sources of communication with the outside world are by the River Gambia and its tributaries, but even after the construction of a road that passes within about twenty kilometres the village remained isolated and showed little interest in the resources, values, and customs of outsiders. The people are mainly Mandinka and they subsist by cultivating the land around the village. They are Muslims who have retained or incorporated aspects of other local beliefs, and the men are polygamous. A few individuals are literate in Arabic, but in this context literacy may not involve much more than a knowledge of the Koran. The village is located in a clearing in the wooded savanna that is characteristic of this part of The Gambia. The people live in mud huts with thatch or corrugated iron roofs. Numerous pathways develop to the fields where cultivation takes place, but these are periodically abandoned as the patterns of land use change. Cultivation and therefore the activities of the villagers is determined by a conspicuously seasonal climate. The long dry season lasts from November to May. There is virtually no rain during this period and the humidity is low, night temperatures may drop to 15° C while during the day it may be extremely hot, especially just before the onset of the rains when temperatures of over 43° C are frequent. The rains begin with thunderstorms and the heaviest rainfall is in August and September. The timing of the rains and the amount of rain that falls varies from year to year as it does in similar savanna environments throughout West Africa. The amount and distribution of rainfall is most important to the productivity of the crops. Most of the agricultural activity is concentrated during the wet season. Cultivation is by hand, mainly with locally made tools, the men being responsible for ground-nuts which are sold for cash, and for grains such as millet, sorghum, and maize, which are consumed locally. The women help in the preparation of the ground for these crops but their main responsibility is the culti-vation of rice in swamps some distance from the village. The rice fields are cleared of weeds at the onset of the rains, planting and transplanting is done in August and September, and the rice ripens and is harvested in November and December. It is likely that the productivity of the rice fields is low as there are no facilities for the control of the numerous pests and diseases that are known to attack the crop in West Africa. Sickness and pregnancy are not regarded as excuses for not cultivating rice and all women who are remotely able to work are forced to do so.

The concentration of heavy agricultural work into a restricted period of the year, together with seasonal changes in the availability of food, has a pronounced effect on the energy budget of the people. From March to May there is little or no work to do, the body weights of the people remain stationary, and their intake and expenditure of energy is low. With the onset of the rains heavy work commences and there is an increase in energy expended, which continues to increase as the rains develop and more and more heavy work becomes necessary. At this time of the year the store of food from the previous harvest is almost exhausted and a seasonal low of available energy is reached at the time when energy expenditure is greatest. This deficit results in a fall in body weight as the tissues of the body are drawn upon. Weight is regained at the beginning of the dry season when food from the harvest becomes available.

A family grows almost all its own food. Rice and millet are the staples, ground-nuts and wild leaves and fruits are used for sauces, and the women and children collect snails and small fish which provide some variation in the diet. Domestic animals such as cattle, goats, and chickens are regarded as status symbols and are killed only on special occasions. Hunting and fishing seem to be unreliable sources of food, although there are presumably plenty of fish avail-able in the river. On the whole food is plentiful in the dry season, but during the wet season when agricultural work is at its peak food is scarce, and in some years cereals are imported from elsewhere.

During the dry season there is rather less risk of disease than during the wet season, but measles and other infections reach epidemic proportions on occasions. A wide variety of infections occur throughout the year, but almost all are more frequent in the wet season when there is the least amount of available food and when agricultural work is most intense. Malaria and other vector-borne diseases are probably mainly transmitted in the wet season when the insect vectors are most abundant. Many of the people have acquired a natural immunity to malaria through repeated exposure when they were children. Filarial infections are common and the children in particular suffer from whooping cough, respiratory and alimentary disorders, and round-worms. Sores are common and persistent. Anaemia seems to be related to the seasonal cycle of malaria, and there is a wide variety of unidentified diseases, possibly attributable to viruses.

As in many Muslim communities ill health and the failure of the crops are usually attributed to the will of Allah. Thomson *et al.* (1968) summarize the attitudes of the Keneba people to illness as follows:

Though tangible causes were given for some diseases (e.g. tsetse flies were thought to cause some paralytic illnesses), most were believed to have a mystical origin. Sepsis was attributed to 'night arrows', evil djinns caused fever, and some types of illness were the results of witchcraft. A 'bad satan' was responsible for most serious or recurrent illnesses, and the specific ethnic influence responsible (e.g. 'Mandinka business') had to be identified in order to effect a cure. . . . Delirium indicated that the Devil was inside the patient and therefore recovery might be undesirable, the people were alarmed that Allah had been cheated by the Devil, and were frightened of the person involved. They reported, apparently with some justification, that the survivors of delirium were often mentally abnormal and unable to fulfil their role in society. Thus, instead of taking curative action, they considered it appropriate to take measures which would ease the sufferer's passage to Paradise. . . . There were many local 'general practitioners' and some 'specialists' in the treatment of illness, in addition to witch doctors and soothsayers. Witch doctors exorcised spirits and destroyed 'bad satans'; the nearest lived about 15 miles away. Soothsayers were more often fortunetellers and herbalists, who prescribed jujus, 'naso' or herbal medicines or rinses. Jujus were usually writings from the Koran and other items enclosed in a leather case and worn round the body. . . . The 'specialists' included a 'paediatrician' and an 'ophthalmologist', both with widespread reputations; a 'physician' who was primarily a herbalist and renowned for his treatment of worms, indigestion and constipation; and several 'surgeons', including a woman who sometimes operated with disastrous consequences, as when she perforated the bowel while incising an abscess.

3 Broken down and decomposing motor cars on an area of grassland in the forest region of Sierra Leone. Wrecked cars are abandoned almost anywhere and the photograph shows a scene becoming increasingly common in tropical Africa.

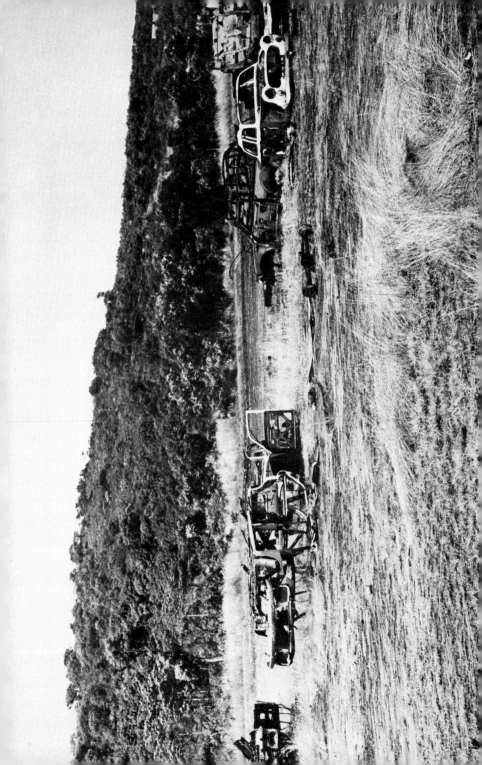

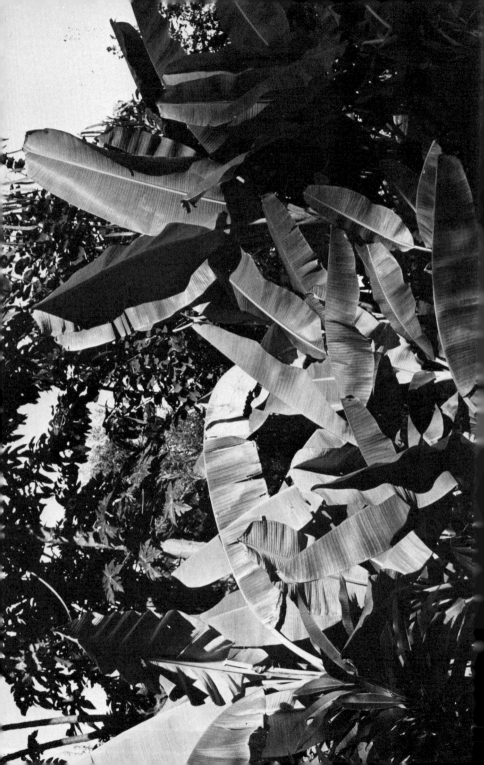

On the whole the people of Keneba have no objection to modern medicine, but they are apt to call in outside help only when local remedies have failed. They are particularly well disposed towards injections, which do not form part of the traditional remedies, although in some parts of Africa they have become incorporated as judged by the rate at which hypodermic syringes disappear from scientific laboratories.

In villages such as Keneba the death rate in children is very high indeed. Children are born into an unhealthy environment, old women often taking part and using magic as a means of facilitating the delivery. They are rather lighter in weight than European babies, but gain weight more quickly, probably because they are breast-fed on demand (Thompson, 1966). But it is not long before they begin to suffer from a wide variety of diseases and 43 per cent of the children born at Keneba die before the age of seven years, mortality being particularly frequent between the ages of nine and fifteen months.

Marsden (1964) has provided a detailed account of the health of babies from birth to eighteen months of age at Sukuta, a Gambian village that is much closer to Bathurst than Keneba and which is provided with a government clinic. Mothers were encouraged to bring their babies to the clinic for regular examination. Of the 152 babies initially registered at the clinic, 32 defaulted within three months and a further 17 subsequently defaulted. Of the initial defaulters, 23 were subsequently traced and six of these are known to have died. Nine of the remaining 103 babies died, two from malaria with severe anaemia, and one each from measles with pneumonia, infective diarrhoea, kwashiorkor, convulsions, lympho-cytic meningitis and anaemia, an unknown fever accompanied by diarrhoea, and as a result of a native medicine. The death rate in this sample is of course much lower than in an area where no doctor is available. The Sukuta babies initially gained weight rapidly, but after the first six months of life the weight gain curve flattened. Weight gain was however irregular and Marsden suggests that the concept of faltering gives a better picture of the situation. Faltering is defined as the failure of a baby to gain more than half a pound (227 g) during a period of three or more months. This allows for correlations to be established between irregular fluctuations in

4 Partially abandoned cultivated land in the forest region, showing bananas growing among native and introduced vegetation. Large areas of Africa are being converted by man into a complex assemblage of crops, weeds, and natural vegetation.

weight and illness. Of the 121 falterings recorded by Marsden, 87 were associated with illness, especially with diarrhoea and malaria, but as he points out, faltering can also occur in the absence of detectable illness or nutritional disturbance. Correlations of this sort are notoriously difficult to interpret and faltering could be the result of the effects of illness or illness could result from faltering, which in turn might be associated with an unknown variable in the environment or in the development of the child. The monthly haemoglobin values in the Sukuta children were similar to those considered to be normal, but were consistently lower, and there was much individual variation. Marsden uses the term 'dipping' to describe brief drops in the haemoglobin level. He found 142 dippings in 76 children during their first eighteen months of life, while in 18 children no dippings were recorded, although it must be stressed that since dipping may occur for very brief periods the monthly assessments that were made would detect only those that happened to coincide with the time of the visit to the clinic. One baby dipped five times and each time this was associated with a sharp attack of malaria. Other workers in tropical Africa have suggested that anaemia is associated with malaria, and the fall in haemoglobin level in the wet season, when malaria is more common, provides additional evidence for this hypothesis. It is interesting that not all babies responded in the same way: this suggests that if malaria is responsible for the fluctuations in haemoglobin level it does not affect all individuals equally.

During the first six months the health of the babies was good. They acquired some immunity to malaria, but after this period their health deteriorated considerably, and during their second wet season they were almost all in poor health. Many more would have died had they not received medical attention, particularly treatment for malaria. The trophozoites of *Plasmodium falciparum*, and sometimes also those of *P. malariae* and *P. ovale*, were found in all but eight of the babies, sometimes more than once. Since babies develop their own immunity to malaria through repeated exposure Marsden suggests that in the Gambian environment anti-malarial drugs should be withheld, except in severe cases. He adopted this policy in his examination of the Sukuta babies and towards the end of the study there was considerable improvement in the response to malaria.

Numerous other infections and conditions were recorded in the Sukuta babies during the eighteen months of study. Some of the more common are shown in Table 10. Many were more frequent in the wet than in the dry season, and the babies suffered much more in the second than in their first wet season of life. Malnutrition was perhaps not as frequent as might have been expected, but it is likely that evidence of malnutrition would not be obvious until after the age of eighteen months. The figures in Table 10 must be treated with caution: skin diseases are far easier to detect than other conditions and are thus probably over-represented. A variety of unidentified fevers occurred, probably caused by viruses. Five babies with convulsions were investigated: two probably had cerebral malaria and one a form of encephalitis. It is likely that cerebral malaria was more frequent as several additional cases of convulsions were reported by the mothers.

The wet season is the worst time of the year for disease in the Gambian villages and in general the health of children was better in the dry season. There is however one disease, measles, that on occasion strikes a heavy blow in the dry season. It varies in intensity from year to year and for reasons that are not fully understood it appears to be a far more serious disease among Africans than Europeans. One possible explanation of this is that many rural Africans are already in poor health when the disease strikes and therefore its effects are more conspicuous. McGregor (1964) has described an epidemic of measles that occurred in Keneba and in the neighbouring villages in the dry season of 1961. The disease is feared by the villagers who believe it comes with the north wind. An eight-year-old child introduced measles into Keneba after returning from an area where the disease was prevalent. The child died soon afterwards and in the meantime the disease had been spread to Jali, a neighbouring village where the first death occurred a little later. By the end of February the disease was spreading rapidly and reached a peak in the middle of March, and then slowly disappeared, the last death being recorded towards the end of April. During the epidemic 62 of the 437 children under 10 years of age in Keneba and Jali died of measles. Table 11 shows the distribution of these deaths by age. The rate of mortality is much higher in the younger children, the death rate in children up to the age of four being more than four times that of the older children. With one exception the adults were not affected and there is evidence that measles had been effectively absent from the area for at least twelve years. The children could not therefore have acquired natural immunity to the disease, but this does not explain the difference between the death rate in the younger and the older children shown in Table 11. McGregor suggests that the younger children were at an age when they would be acquiring immunity to a variety of other diseases, notably malaria, yellow fever, poliomyelitis, and diphtheria, and as a result they were less able to withstand the measles virus and resulting secondary infections.

The most striking effect of this epidemic of measles is that it disrupted the normal seasonal pattern of mortality among the children of the area. Table 12 shows the monthly distribution of deaths at Jali in each year from 1957 to 1963. The year 1961 stands out from the rest because of the conspicuously higher mortality in February–April through measles. In most years there are more deaths in the wet season, but 1961 provided an exception to the usual pattern. The epidemic also affected the subsequent pattern of births, as many women became pregnant soon after losing their child and there was later an unusual number of births which in turn exposed more children than usual to the hardship of the wet season.

There is increasing evidence that measles is one of the most severe diseases of children in Africa. It is one of the main causes of blindness, although it seems that blindness is more frequent than it need be because of the use of harmful local remedies. McGregor (1964) compares the impact of measles in the two Gambian villages in 1961 with the impact of the disease on the population of England and Wales in the same year. In 1961 there were 763 465 reported cases of measles in England and Wales of which only 152 (0·02 per cent) were fatal. In Keneba and Jali with a combined population of 1400, measles killed 62 people, or 4·4 per cent of the population, and 14·2 per cent of the children under 10 years of age.

Measles is an example of only one epidemic that can sweep through a rural population. Such epidemics as this have manifold effects on the birth patterns, availability of women as manual labourers during the cultivating season, and on the role of local practitioners of medicine. They can also reinforce religious beliefs and strengthen the already strong associations between the people, the environment, and the gods.

One possible cause of the high death rate among children suffering from measles in tropical Africa is that the children are much more in direct contact with other individuals than is normal in Europe. Thus a young child is usually carried about all day on its mother's back and if the mother is working in the fields the child is exposed to the risk of infection from others. Another possible reason is that the children are already suffering from other diseases and in particular may have insufficient protein to eat. It is extremely difficult to separate the reasons for the severity of diseases such as measles among African children. Morley (1967) in offering a practical approach to problems of child health in the tropics suggests that since in Africa many children suffer from diseases while they are younger than European children they are consequently likely to suffer more severely. Table 13 shows the average ages at which children from different parts of the world are affected by two diseases, measles and whooping cough. The average age of infection for both diseases is nearly twice as high in Britain and North America as it is in Africa. Morley feels that the high mortality from whooping cough in African children is mainly because they contract the disease while much younger than children in developed countries. As far as measles is concerned he feels that environmental effects are of more importance, in particular the state of nutrition of the child.

The long-term study of rural children in Nigeria reported by Morley (1963) may be compared with Marsden's study of children in The Gambia. The people are mainly Yoruba cultivators living in rather dense populations in what was the rain forest belt of Western Nigeria. Yams, maize, and cassava are the main food crops and cocoa is grown as a cash crop. The children are carried about on the backs of the mothers for the first two years and this Morley considers is generally advantageous as the child receives constant attention and feeding on demand, but as mentioned earlier it may also facilitate the transmission of disease. Before the establishment of a medical service for children under five years of age, over 50 per cent of the children died before they were four years of age. This figure includes stillbirths which, however, were not particularly frequent. In the 1–4 age group the death rate was sixty times higher than among comparable children in England and Wales. The main causes of death were disease and malnutrition, many children dying of multiple conditions, diarrhoea, pneumonia, malnutrition, malaria, and measles being the more important. The establishment of a clinic after 1957 substantially reduced the death rate, but the results were less spectacular than might have been expected because of an outbreak of measles, considered by Morley to be the deadliest of all diseases in West African children. Local practices associated with child care were not in general thought to be harmful, except possibly clitoridectomy which may lead to much loss of blood.

Mortality among children in rural Africa is high and from this it follows that those that become adults will have acquired a certain amount of immunity to some of the more important diseases. But even so the state of health of many adults is poor which in turn means that the capacity for heavy work is low. Adults are less likely to suffer from malnutrition than children because they are no longer growing, but many individuals are infected with a wide variety of parasites which have a debilitating effect and reduce working efficiency. Large families are the rule and there are virtually no attempts to limit family size, although children may be somewhat spaced out as a result of taboos that forbid intercourse while the mother is still feeding a baby from the breast.

One group of adults in particular seem especially liable to ill health. These are the migrant labourers whose work is seasonal and dependent on when and where certain crops are grown on large plantations. While they are working they earn some money and indeed are attracted to this way of life by the short-term benefits it seems to offer. They rarely consider saving and when the season is over they usually have insufficient money to return to their own homes. Because of their way of life in which they are unable to fall back on the extended family system of the villages, they suffer more from malnutrition and disease than other adults. Giel and Van Luijk (1967) have described the plight of daily labourers in a coffee-growing province in Ethiopia as follows:

Every morning of the week all sorts of people adorn the steps of the provincial hospital in Kaffa-province, Ethiopia, waiting to be treated for their ailments. One group, however, strikes the eye as being particularly miserable and despairing. These are the daily labourers, the coolies or *kenseratenja* as they call themselves. The leftovers of the coffee season who at one time converged upon Jimma from all over Ethiopia to earn a good wage. Now they are in rags, and on closer examination they appear to be covered with lice. They sit and lie on the porches of the hospital, sometimes for days on end. Aside from their personal misery, they seem to be a hazard to the community as far as public health is concerned.

Giel and Van Luijk examined 170 of these daily labourers and compared their health with that of 599 residents of the area. The labourers could buy meals cheaply, but often had insufficient money to pay for an adequate amount of food and on some days had no food at all. Whenever possible they had three meals a day usually consisting of three small pancakes or two of these with a piece of bread, a quantity of the spicy local sauce, and one or two cups of tea. The sauce contained very little meat and they hardly ever ate fruit or vegetables. It must be assumed that besides a lack of quantity of food they also received inadequate amounts of protein and vitamins. Table 14 shows the frequency of the diseases that were found in the 170 labourers and for comparison the frequency of the same diseases in the sample of people resident in the area. It was estimated that 58 per cent of the labourers were suffering from infectious diseases that could be prevented while among the residents the comparable figure was 22 per cent. The diseases listed in Table 14 as being of unknown origin were probably made up mainly of malaria which could not be positively detected, but possibly also typhus and relapsing fever. Venereal diseases were six times as frequent among the labourers as among the residents, but this may be partly because the latter included children. Severe malnutrition was more frequent among the residents and again this can be attributed to the presence of children in the sample who are much more likely to suffer from severe malnutrition.

As in The Gambia the incidence of malaria in Ethiopia is higher during the wet than during the dry season and indeed during the wet season malaria may be almost universal, although considered by itself it probably does not account for a significant adult mortality.

The picture of morbidity obtained from this sample of migrant labourers is probably representative of people in this category throughout Africa. The advantage of village life is that the extended family system is able to cope with sickness and a considerable amount of help is provided by relatives and friends. This help may take the form of looking after children and also of providing food and shelter for adults.

The visitor to Africa will frequently remark on the number of adults that can be seen sitting around in villages apparently doing nothing. What is not fully appreciated is that many of these people are suffering and have been suffering for a long time from one or more debilitating diseases and that their diet is nutritionally inadequate. There are in rural areas few jobs that earn money and the only work possible is that of producing sufficient food to keep going. The weather is usually hot during the day and in humid areas manual work is by no means easy, even for a healthy person. Such work that is done is usually concentrated in the early morning and in the evening when it is a little cooler. The somewhat fatalistic outlook adopted is not difficult to understand and exists in European societies as well as in Africa.

A visitor from a developed country may not be aware that there exist in most areas of Africa well-tried and traditional ways of diagnosing and remedying ill health and indisposition. The absence of familiar medicines and medical facilities does not necessarily mean that the condition is being neglected; throughout tropical Africa people have for generations used plants and plant derivatives, and less frequently special extracts from animals, as remedies for ill health. This of course is not peculiar to Africa: people throughout the world favour local remedies and only recently have these been replaced by modern medicine. Not only are these remedies directed against specific symptoms that are recognized but also against illness that has supposedly been caused by a person's misdemeanours; that is to say a certain remedy may be necessary if one falls ill because one has stolen from another person or if one has in any way lived dishonestly. An incredible number of species of plants are utilized in this way, and in addition are used for the treatment of sickness in domestic animals, as aphrodisiacs, and as poisons. Many plants contain in their tissues chemical compounds that are toxic to animals that eat them, others contain compounds that are not exactly toxic but which act as repellents. It is these properties of plants that are being exploited in the local remedies.

The use of plant extracts as a cure for human illness often involves the use of magic and sometimes leads to elaborate ceremonies in which many people take part. Cures for madness are especially complex and besides the administration of the appropriate medicine by the proper authority there is usually a lengthy ceremony during which the evil spirit that is supposedly within the victim is exorcized. Madness is often considered as a punishment by the gods for some wrong the victim may have committed and so the appropriate cure is given only after the victim has suffered for what is considered to be a suitable period of time. It is widely believed that only certain individuals can remove the evil spirit and sometimes a man has to be sent long distances in order to receive the correct treatment from the right person.

Some of the plants that are used to cure illness are known to contain chemical compounds that are likely to be effective for certain illnesses. Thus many plant compounds can initiate an emetic reaction which is sometimes desirable if poisoning is suspected. In recent years chemists and botanists have combined to study the indigenous uses of plants, but the work thus far has involved mainly the identification of the compounds present in the plants rather than extensive testing (which would present special problems) of the values of the compounds as cures for illness. Moreover it could be reasonably argued that the compounds themselves are unlikely to work as efficiently if administered under the sterile conditions of the laboratory and without the aid of medicine men and magic. Numerous accounts have been published on the uses of plants as a cure for illness. They are based mainly on hearsay evidence gathered by botanists and others from translated verbal accounts given to them by people in rural areas. Chemists investigating the properties of these plants have often confirmed the presence of compounds that could conceivably be effective in curing certain illnesses. The detailed account of the useful plants of West Africa (Dalziel, 1937) provides a wealth of information on the uses of plants as medicines, as also does the book on the woody plants of Ghana (Irvine, 1961). Space does not permit a summary of the contents of these and other similar works, and I shall therefore confine this discussion to the uses of one particular plant.

The plant I have chosen is *Calotropis procera*, a milkweed

belonging to the Asclepiadaceae, a family of plants renowned for the presence of cardiac glycosides (heart poisons) in the tissues. The plant is common throughout the savanna of tropical Africa, growing to a height of several metres. It has been planted in and around the coastal towns of West Africa, possibly by people from the savanna who have moved into the towns to seek employment and who at the same time require a ready supply of the plant.[1] The extent to which the milky latex of *Calotropis procera* is poisonous is not fully known, but there is some evidence that it is lethal only if taken in large doses. In various parts of Africa the latex is used as an arrow poison, but possibly only when mixed with other plant poisons. It is rubbed on the skin as a cure for rheumatism and on the chest as a cure for a cough. The juice from warmed leaves is placed in the nose, causing sneezing and relief from headache and catarrh. In Northern Nigeria and Ghana it is used for conjunctivitis, ringworm, and sores in the mouths of children, and a piece of wool soaked in latex is sometimes placed on a decaying tooth. In the Sudan gonorrhoea is treated by injecting a solution into the rectum. The latex may also be used for infanticide and to procure abortion, but in Ghana a barren woman is treated by local application of fresh leaves pulverized with red peppers, and if labour is difficult a poultice of the leaves may be applied to the abdomen. In Northern Nigeria the dried leaves are burnt and the smoke inhaled as a cure for asthma, while the root is used in the treatment of syphilis. One method of treating syphilis demands that the leaves be pounded in water in which corn has been soaked, and then after the liquid has been left standing for a few days it is drunk in large quantities causing vomiting and diarrhoea with discharge, which, it is believed, represents the spawn of the disease. The bark of the root is said to be useful as a cure for dysentery and when pulverized is added to soup and taken to relieve stomach upsets. Extracts from the bark of the root are also supposed to encourage lactation. In Senegal the root is used in the treatment of leprosy and charcoal from the roots is rubbed on skin eruptions. The aphrodisiac properties of the roots

[1] Many other plants of reputed medicinal value have been introduced from the savanna into the forest region of West Africa. The importance of such introductions in the present distribution of plants is a topic that seems to have been neglected by plant geographers.

are recognized in Senegal, and throughout Africa various parts of the plant or extracts mixed with those of other plants are used to cure diseases in domestic animals. Numerous other uses of a non-medicinal nature have been recorded, and in Senegal the plant is placed over doorways to prevent witchcraft.

Calotropis procera is just one example of a plant with multiple medicinal uses. An enormous variety of plants is used in a similar way. Many wild plants are also used as a means of flavouring sauces that are consumed with carbohydrate staples, and it is likely that the incorporation of such plants in the diet may be medicinal in origin.

Most of the people living in rural areas have become adapted to changes brought about by the introduction of crops and domestic animals from elsewhere. Many introductions occurred a long time ago: cattle have been present in Africa for several thousand years, and many of the carbohydrate staple foods were brought in hundreds of years ago from other tropical regions of the world. Most rural people are cultivators or pastoralists, but there are a few remaining groups who have been relatively unaffected by the introduction of cultivation and pastoralism. The continued existence of these people is threatened because the habitats in which they live are likely to be destroyed by the expanding populations of cultivators and pastoralists. In addition their special needs are rarely considered by administrators and politicians. The two main groups of such people are the pygmies of the Congo forests and the bushmen of the Kalahari Desert.

The Mbuti pygmies form a discrete population living in the Ituri Forest in the north-eastern part of the Congo. There are only about 40 000 of them and they are essentially hunters and gatherers, dependent almost entirely on the natural products of the forest. In the same area there are cultivators who on the whole fear and despise the forest, and whose main interest is to cut down the trees and plant crops. The pygmies understandably regard the cultivators as a threat to their existence, for unlike the cultivators they make no attempt to control (and therefore destroy) their environment. Turnbull (1961) suggests that there is a kind of mutually acceptable apartheid between the pygmies and the cultivators and that although there is some trade between them there is little interest in each other's affairs. The life of the pygmies is closely adapted to the special conditions of the forest, and it is therefore not astonishing that they regard non-forest people with suspicion and hostility. And yet it appears that the forest will be destroyed and Turnbull suggests that the problem of accommodating the Mbuti in a non-forest environment without destroying them is insurmountable. The Ituri consists of an extensive area of primary forest with an enormous diversity of species of trees, plants, and animals. The climate is rather uniform all the year round and the Mbuti, who are known to have inhabited the forest for at least 5000 years, are rarely short of food, and probably suffer less from malnutrition than the nearby cultivators. Only one main road cuts through the forest and it is along this road that the cultivators have settled. The forest itself is inhabited only by the pygmies who live in rather small bands. They regard themselves as the children of the forest and according to Turnbull they refer to it as 'mother' or 'father', rationalizing that the forest like their own mother and father provides food, shelter, warmth, and affection. They hunt the forest animals, but have not exploited the fish that abound in the streams. They collect a wide variety of invertebrates, including the large achatinid snails, the larvae of moths, and termites. The women especially are the gatherers and they collect mushrooms, roots, berries, and nuts, moving from species to species as the season changes. All of these activities require expert knowledge of what is edible and what is poisonous. The rewards from hunting and gathering may vary with the season and also from year to year, but the enormous diversity of plant and animal life ensures an adequate food supply all the year round. The social organization of the Mbuti pygmies is highly adapted to the most efficient ways of hunting and gathering: bands are not too large and not too small, different bands of hunters know each other well and the interactions between them are friendly. The size of the band may be adjusted to fluctuations in the available food, particularly to the availability of game animals. The society is highly democratic and there are no chiefs, elders, priests, or other specialists who might exert an authoritarian influence; the opinions of all members are sought and individuals with specialized knowledge receive considerable attention in the proper circumstances. Turnbull points out that their ultimate loyalty is to the forest, the provider of all that is good. If anyone upsets the smooth running of a band it is customary to remind him that it is the forest that he is really upsetting.

The pygmies are therefore well adjusted to their environment and have been in this position without outside interference for many generations. But the forest is now threatened by exploitation from outsiders whom the pygmies despise and distrust. Turnbull thinks that they are ill-adapted to life outside the forest and that when removed from their own environment they tend to die of sunstroke and disorders of the stomach. Their future is not bright as they will soon have to cope with people who want to alter the environment to suit themselves rather than adjust to the special conditions of the forest.

The Kalahari Desert in south-western Africa is a vast area covered with dry bush and dominated by well-dispersed and often very large baobab trees. For most of the year the climate is hot and dry, although in the winter night temperatures are low and water may freeze. There are three months of rain and during the rains the desert is alive with flowering plants, and there is plenty of standing water. In the dry season there is no surface water and the landscape is extremely dry and barren. In this area of Africa live the bushmen, between thirty and fifty thousand of them, of unknown ethnic origin, but almost certainly unrelated to the negroids. Like the pygmies they are well adjusted to the special environment in which they live and are highly suspicious and distrustful of outsiders. The similarity between the two groups of people is striking: both live in environments that are not attractive to other people, both are considerably smaller and paler than the negroids, and both are organized into hunting and gathering bands, the men the hunters and the women the gatherers. But the bushmen, unlike the pygmies, live in an environment that is hard and seasonal: they are often hungry and the bands have to travel from place to place seeking food. Their suspicion of strangers is indicated by the various names they have for other people all of which suggest an element of distrust. The bushmen are hard to find, especially as they have no permanent homes, and they are remarkably good at concealing themselves in the desert. When they encounter outsiders they are apt to be submissive, and call themselves 'the harmless people', which is the title given to an informative book on their ways and customs (Thomas, 1960).

The bushmen have an extensive knowledge of the desert plants especially those with underground roots that hold water and which consequently are much sought after in the dry season when water is scarce. Desert and arid savanna regions of Africa contain numerous species of Cucurbitaceae, and the bushmen gather the melonlike fruits for the water they contain, and also use them as containers for water. The Kalahari is unlikely to be exploited in the near future as the climate is unsuitable for crops and there is not enough vegetation and water for cattle. The bushmen have in the past suffered at the hands of the Europeans and the Bantu-speakers and their present restricted distribution is probably largely the result of outside pressures. Their future is uncertain, and as more and more of them leave their own society and join the negroids their traditional way of life will disintegrate. Like the pygmies they have learnt to live with their environment without destroying it, but in the modern world this way of life no longer seems acceptable.

I have tried in this chapter to provide an account of the lives of people in the rural areas of Africa, indicating so far as possible the numerous hazards to everyday existence. It is hoped that an understanding of some of the problems confronted by the rural people will provide some basis for future programmes of development. Almost everywhere the rapidly expanding human population is altering the natural environment and the few groups of people who are living in equilibrium with their environment are threatened with extinction by the activities of the cultivators and the pastoralists. The infant mortality rates described are extremely high but undoubtedly the means will be found to improve the chances of survival of the children and this in turn will generate what is likely to be a major ecological crisis as the resulting population increases gather momentum.

CHAPTER 4

Life and Death in Urban Africa

As in all parts of the world the towns and cities of tropical Africa have two important characteristics: they are expanding in size at a phenomenal rate, and they attract people from all walks of life and of diverse ethnic origin. Large towns lack the social cohesion of the villages and the plight of the poor is in many ways more striking: an individual in distress has fewer possibilities of seeking help from relations and friends than in a village in which the extended family system operates well. Some African towns are dominated by a single ethnic group, Ibadan by the Yoruba, for example, but there is usually also a large minority from numerous other ethnic groups. People in different ethnic groups tend to keep to themselves: jobs and opportunities tend to be awarded on a strictly ethnic basis, which although tolerated creates individual dissatisfaction, especially when so many people are unemployed. The commerce of many of the larger African towns is dominated by Asians, particularly by Indians in East Africa and by Lebanese in West Africa. Much of the business is controlled by Europeans. There have been moves on the part of governments to prohibit non-citizens from indulging in certain kinds of commercial activities. Thus in Sierra Leone non-citizens are not allowed to sell rice, matches, umbrellas, and a number of other items. These laws have been passed in the hope that local people will take a more active part in the retail trade, but whether this will be possible remains to be seen. In some instances commercial firms operated by non-citizens have had to close because of the new laws, much to the annoyance of the richer citizens who like to patronize supermarkets and well-appointed shops. Commercial enterprises have also had to close because they have been unable to obtain work permits for non-citizens and because of large-scale stealing by their junior employees.

Almost all the capital cities in tropical Africa have an airport open to international traffic, a television station, and a university. Almost all have better medical and school facilities than the rural areas, but health and school education have been less lucky in receiving funds for improvements than universities and airports. Educated Africans prefer to live in towns, and those sent to try their skills in rural areas spend much of their time trying to obtain a job in or near the capital city, relying heavily on the influence that a relative in a high position may be able to use to facilitate this. As a result most of the teachers and doctors in the towns and cities are Africans, while many of those in rural areas are Europeans or Asians.

The establishment of a town depends on the availability of resources in the area. Large towns develop in areas where resources are most available and especially where communications are good. This explains why many of the larger African towns are located on rivers or by the coast. The availability of fresh water is possibly one of the most important factors determining the establishment and subsequent development of a town. The size and dispersion of towns is thus very similar to the size and dispersion of nesting colonies of birds: large colonies occur close together in areas where resources are good, and small well-scattered colonies occur in areas where resources are poor. Some of the large towns of Africa were already well established when the Europeans first arrived. The Yoruba in particular tended to settle in large groups in Western Nigeria, and unlike most people in Africa they were to a large extent pre-adapted to the European concept of a town.

The city of Freetown was established in 1792 when over a thousand freed slaves were brought from Nova Scotia. There had been some earlier settlement of the area by people known as the 'black poor' who had been brought from London, but these were scattered after the settlement was attacked by people from inland. Various additional groups of freed slaves arrived from the Americas and from captured slaving ships from around 1800 and throughout the next thirty years. In 1808 there were 2000 people in Freetown and by 1833 there were 10 000. During this period adult mortality rates, and presumably also infant deaths, were very high. Indeed Sierra Leone was known at one time as the white man's grave, a name that even today it has had some difficulty in living down. By 1870 there were 20 000 people in Freetown and the population reached 33 000 by 1914. The 1930 census revealed 55 000 people and by 1963 there were about 128 000, indicating that the city had doubled its population in about thirty years. The rapid increase in population size is partly the result of improved health and partly a consequence of migration into the city by people hoping to earn a living. Hence not only has the city grown in size but it has also changed in ethnic composition. The creoles are now in the minority while the Temne and the Mende from the interior of the country are now extremely numerous. There is every reason to suppose that the present rate of expansion of the population will continue, indeed the rate itself shows signs of increasing.

Freetown was established as a result of the British policy of abolishing slavery and it later grew because of its strategic position in terms of trade with Europe. Most large towns in tropical Africa were not established by freed slaves but grew from existing villages in response to the trading demands of the Europeans. Towns grew most rapidly in areas where raw materials could be exploited and successfully transported for overseas shipment, and also where there was a need to centralize the administrative control of the territory.

Literacy is more common in the towns than in the villages and many people have access to newspapers and radios. Possibly as a consequence there is more knowledge of the nutritional value of food, and except among the very poor, examples of severe malnutrition are less frequent. A wide variety of food is available in the markets and although there is sometimes a seasonal scarcity of a staple food there is rarely a real shortage, provided there is money to buy it. The diversity of goods for sale in the markets is astonishing. Besides the staple foods there are all kinds of cultivated and gathered delicacies that may be used in sauces or for flavouring. Near the coast and around large lakes and rivers dried and smoked fish are often available in quantity, and live chickens can be bought almost everywhere. The extent to which wild foods are marketed varies between ethnic groups, but in many areas it is possible to buy land snails, various insects, and even rodents. Outsiders, including the charitable organizations, have sometimes drawn attention to the sale of such items as evidence of food scarcity, but this is erroneous as many people like these delicacies which form an expected part of the diet of even the most affluent people.

The staple crops are grown in rural areas some distance from the big centres of population and nowadays are sent to town by road. In some areas insufficient food is grown in the rural areas for export to the towns and the staples have to be supplemented by imports from overseas. Thus in Freetown where rice is the staple food there is periodically a local scarcity and citizens anxiously await the arrival of the next ship bringing rice from North America, Burma, or even Egypt. The periodic scarcity of rice is not because it is impossible to grow more but because the rural people tend to grow enough for themselves and do not worry too much about the sale of rice to others. In Sierra Leone the Chinese have demonstrated that the yield of rice from an area of land can be increased several times if proper care is taken and if the crop is harvested and planted at the correct time of year.

It is difficult to be certain but it is likely that the health of people in the towns is in general better than that of people in rural areas. Death is not more or less inevitable if a person contracts a serious disease because it is possible to obtain medical treatment at the hospitals, which although usually poorly equipped and under-staffed, are able to provide the sort of service that can effectively prevent a seriously ill person from dying. The birth rate in towns appears to be as high as elsewhere, but the survival of children is better, although low by comparison with Europe. The numbers of children to be seen on the streets is impressive: in Freetown the streets are almost completely blocked when the schools let the children out in the afternoon; there are children everywhere and many of them appear to be in good health.

Almost all of the diseases characteristic of the African countryside affect the people in towns, and epidemics are frequent and sometimes devastating. To these diseases must be added some other causes of injury and death which thus far have not been so important in the villages. All of them are of a social nature.

Everywhere the standard of driving is low. In Uganda it is esti-mated that the road accident rate is about six times as high as it is in Europe. Most of the people killed in road accidents are the drivers and their passengers, the most affluent people in the community, many of them occupying key positions, and the high death rate thus removes a considerable number of doctors, teachers, government officials, and others in important positions. Some governments are becoming worried about the high accident rates on the roads. In Nigeria it has been recognized that drugs are often taken by long-distance drivers and although the importance of drugs on the accident rate is not known it is thought to be considerable.

The brewing and distillation of alcoholic drinks is one of the few industries that appears to be flourishing in the towns. People with money tend to drink heavily but the extent to which alcoholism is a major hazard to health appears to be unexplored. Drinking and driving are strongly correlated and it would seem likely that an additional cause of high road accident rates is drunkenness.

In addition to the medical facilities offered by government and private hospitals there are a number of other ways in which an individual can receive medical treatment or can treat himself. Important government officials and politicians are frequently sent to Europe for medical treatment, sometimes going for no more than a routine check-up. At the other extreme rural people who have moved into the towns seeking jobs but who have neither the money nor the knowledge to obtain proper treatment have two possibilities open to them. One is to buy one or more of the numerous patent medicines (which are cheap) that are available almost everywhere and are widely advertised as a cure to common illnesses. These are marketed by European firms who find a ready sale in Africa for products which they would have difficulty selling in their own country for fear of a public investigation. All kinds of medicines and instant cures are advertised. One common brand sold in West Africa is said to cure backache and kidney troubles. As everyone experiences backache from time to time the product enjoys considerable popularity. A dose of the medicine turns the urine green, thus proving its effectiveness, and of course the backache goes away, which it would have done anyway. These medicines are undoubtedly convincing to people used to village specialists that prescribe all sorts of cures accompanied by the appropriate magic and ceremony. Many wage earners in the lower income brackets spend sizeable proportions of their money on remedies to minor ailments, real or otherwise. The situation may be compared with the sale of cosmetics in Europe, many of which are frequently claimed to have almost magical properties.

Mulago Hospital at Kampala in Uganda is a university teaching and research hospital with excellent modern equipment and highly skilled scientists and doctors attached to its staff. It is possible to obtain medical attention at this hospital that compares favourably with the best available in Europe. And yet within sight of the hospital witch doctors perform operations on young women unable to conceive children, often with disastrous consequences, and in Kampala itself all sorts of magic aids to health are sold by specialists. Near the hospital there is a large roost of the fruit bat, *Eidolon helvum*, and these bats are collected from time to time by individuals who require the blood to concoct a medicine for a specific ailment.

The most important potential threat to urban health in tropical Africa is probably associated with the quality of the water available for human consumption. Until recently many densely populated towns had an inadequate water supply. This has been remedied in some places by the construction of dams and the introduction of piped water, but even now the majority of the people obtain their water from communal pumps, sites that have been long recognized as sources of major outbreaks of disease in Europe and elsewhere. The extent to which water-borne diseases affect the health of urban populations is not known, but as human numbers continue to rise and there is an increasing demand for water it would seem likely that the risk of epidemics will grow. With a few exceptions most of the dams that have been constructed recently near large towns cannot be expected to provide an adequate supply of water for more than about a decade.

As is well-known, people in European towns lived under appalling conditions at the time of the industrial revolution. The large factories that developed were extremely unhealthy and the death rates among people that moved from rural areas to find work in the centres of developing industry were extremely high, particularly among the young people. This situation has of course changed as the result of social reform and the invention of efficient and labour saving machines. The industries in the towns of industrial Europe are based on raw materials obtained from elsewhere and in the last 50 to 100 years an increasing amount of these raw materials has been obtained from tropical countries, including many of those of Africa. These raw materials include renewable and non-renewable resources, the latter being mostly obtained by mining operations of one sort or another. The rapid development of mining in Africa over the past fifty years has given rise to numerous large or medium-sized towns whose populations are dependent on the job opportunities offered by mining. The health of the people in these mining towns has until recently been a matter of conjecture. It had been thought that the health of the people was poor (World Health Organization, 1960), but no evidence was available to substantiate this belief. Mills (1967a) appears to have been the first to investigate the health of people in a mining area compared with the health of the surrounding rural population. Earlier than this some studies had been made of urban populations but comparative information on the surrounding rural areas was not obtained. Mills' work was carried out at Lunsar in Sierra Leone and the account that follows is based on his study.

The town of Lunsar is about 120 km east of Freetown and is located on a plain covered with secondary bush which at one time was rain forest. Two large mountains containing iron ore emerge from the plain. At the start of mining operations in 1929 there were only about seven houses at Lunsar, but with the introduction of mining equipment and the establishment of a railway link people started to move into the area, including both miners and tradesmen who expected to sell goods to the relatively affluent miners. In 1959 there was a population of about 10 000 drawn chiefly from the surrounding rural areas, and Mills was thus able to compare the health of the urban population with that of the rural population. He selected four villages located between eleven and thirty-two kilometres from Lunsar to compare with the urban population of Lunsar. A total of 1010 people from the villages and 954 from the town were examined. Table 15 shows the ethnic composition of the two samples. The area around Lunsar is predominantly Temne and nearly all the people in the villages belong to this group. Temne also outnumber all the other groups put together in Lunsar, but there is a higher frequency of the other groups. Thus there are no creoles in the villages and their presence in Lunsar is undoubtedly because they have moved in to work in the offices associated with the mining. The higher frequency of Fula in Lunsar is because these people are known for their abilities as petty traders, a niche for which there should be some demand in a mining town. Nearly three-quarters of the people in the villages were born where they lived, but only just over a quarter of those in Lunsar were born there. Both the ethnic composition and the place of birth indicate that the Lunsar population contains a far higher proportion of immigrants than the population of the villages. The living conditions in Lunsar and the villages differ considerably. Many of the houses in Lunsar have corrugated iron roofs while in the villages most of the roofs are of thatch and are more 'traditional'. The Lunsar houses are more overcrowded than those in the villages with an average of 16 persons per house as against 10 per house in the villages. The village people obtain their water from streams and rivers, and in the dry season there is a relatively small flow of water and the streams become muddy and contaminated. About three-quarters of the people in Lunsar make use of a piped supply of water which is available for 2–4 hours a day. In both populations the danger of infection from water-borne diseases is considerable, but possibly the situation in the villages is worse because of the unreliability of the water supply in the dry season.

In Table 16 the morbidity rates in the two samples are compared. The extent to which individuals, positive for malaria, onchocerciasis, and nutritional deficiency, were actually suffering from these diseases is variable, but the figures may be taken as an indication of the difference between people in the urban and the rural environment. As shown, malaria is much more prevalent in the villages, but the biggest difference is the high rate of nutritional disorders in the villages compared with the town. The figures for onchocerciasis are about the same in the two samples. Nutritional deficiencies arise primarily through a shortage of protein and it seems likely that the availability of money to the people in the town went some way to rectify this deficiency as they would be able to buy a wider range of foods. Almost all the other pathological conditions recorded by Mills occurred more frequently in the villages than in the town. Birth rates are somewhat lower in the town and average family size a little smaller. This together with the fact that the mining company provides an efficient health service for its 2400 employees and their families and that 26 per cent of the males in the town work for the company and are entitled to the benefits it offers, results in the town population being considerably healthier than the rural population.

The high rate of onchocerciasis found in the area (Table 16) prompted an examination of the Europeans working for the mining company. Of the 116 European staff and their families, 73 were screened for onchocerciasis and none was found to be positive (Mills, 1967b). Onchocerciasis is transmitted by a fly, *Simulium*, and although the Europeans were constantly exposed to bites from the flies and the densities of the fly were the same in the areas frequented by both the African and the European population, the Europeans were free from the disease. Mills suggests that this is because Europeans have better living conditions and are less tolerant towards flies, often taking preventive measures against being bitten while at work, at home, and at places of recreation, particularly at the swimming pool to which they are most partial.

Mills' study indicates that improved health facilities in a town can to some extent decrease the general morbidity of the population. Whether the pattern discovered at Lunsar is widespread remains to be shown.

CHAPTER 5

The Ecology of Cultivation

During the middle and late Pleistocene the people that lived in Africa were busily engaged in making tools and weapons from stone, and later on from metal. These tools and weapons, especially various forms of hand axe, have been found throughout Africa except in the forested regions of the west and centre. There is abundant evidence that until relatively recently what is now the Sahara Desert was covered with vegetation and that there were more people living there than now. It also seems that the invention of a particular tool or weapon was quickly followed by the spread of its use over a vast region, suggesting that there was a considerable movement of at least some segments of the population or that information about the invention of a new implement spread quickly. The tools appear to have been used mainly for hunting and gathering, but it is felt that conflicts between rival groups of people may often have led to war and that many of the so-called tools are in reality weapons. The apparent absence of implements from the more humid parts of tropical Africa suggests either that there were few or no people or that such people that did exist were isolated from the cultural developments that were occurring in the savanna. Some anthropologists contend that tools would be less in demand in the humid regions where food could be more easily obtained than in the savanna, which is seasonally more demanding and thus possibly more stimulating to the human imagination.

In Africa, the cultivation of plants for food and the domestication of animals started in Egypt about 8000 years ago and rapidly spread across North Africa and into what is now the Sahara Desert. About 2000 years later cultivation and the keeping of domestic animals, especially cattle, was widespread throughout this area, but the habit did not spread into sub-Saharan Africa until much later. Clark (1964) suggests that the failure of cultivation to spread into tropical and southern Africa was because of the wealth of wild foods in the area. Thus in effect he is suggesting that there was no need for the development of cultivation, even though with the knowledge of tool-making that existed, this would have been a perfectly feasible enterprise. The Sahara began to dry up about 4500 years ago and this is believed to have forced the cultivators and the pastoralists south into the tropical savanna. The plants they were cultivating were cereals, such as barley and wheat, which are difficult to grow in a tropical climate, and as the people moved south it would seem that they must have experimented with edible wild plants, occasionally finding among them species that were suitable for cultivation. Thus from about 4000 years ago onwards a number of indigenous tropical African plants were cultivated in the northern savanna. One of these was sorghum, and it was probably about this time that the first genetic changes were induced in the wild plant by selective breeding and cultivation. Murdock (1959, 1960) and others have suggested that the people around the headwaters of the Niger independently developed agriculture, and among the several crops they domesticated, sorghum was the most important. But the bulk of the evidence suggests that agriculture was brought south across the Sahara by people who necessarily had to move because of the change in climate. Cultivators were well established in Northern Nigeria between 2000 and 4000 years ago, and during this time metal tools began to replace those made of stone. Cultivators also reached Ethiopia and the Kenya Rift Valley area about 4000 years ago, but there is little evidence of the spread of cultivation further south into the forest region until much later.

During the early phases of the introduction of agriculture into tropical Africa it is likely that the human population was rather small and well dispersed, but about 2000 years ago there appears to have been something of a minor population explosion which heralded the extensive movements of the Bantu-speaking people. This event may have considerably speeded up the development of agriculture, especially as by this time the use of iron implements was becoming more widespread. But it is equally likely that the increasing dependence on agriculture itself generated the increase in human numbers. It is probable that the first introductions of food plants directly from Asia took place soon after the population increase, and the development of subsistence agriculture of the kind seen today in tropical Africa can be assumed to have started. As discussed in Chapter 1, the origin and spread of the negroids is one of the unsolved problems in the early ecological history of modern man in Africa. But whatever their origins it would appear that as they spread they took with them the beginnings of agriculture.

Compared with other parts of the world cultivation started late in tropical Africa. For hundreds of generations man had hunted and gathered and Allan (1965), discussing the early development of agriculture in Africa, makes the point that although man had been present in Africa for a very long time, 'for all but a fraction of this time there is no trace of any higher form of exploitation than the "robber" economy of savagery'. This may be so, but from the point of view of population ecology, early man achieved a better balance with his environment than the present-day cultivators who tend to destroy rather than rationally exploit the available resources. It could also be questioned whether hunting and gathering are savage occupations: both require considerable skill, in many ways more skill than is required by the cultivator who is simply using the results of trial and error selection of crops. The chief effect of cultivation is that the carrying capacity of the land is increased and it is becoming questionable as to whether this represents an advance. Hunting and gathering are primitive in the sense that they occurred earlier than cultivation in man's cultural evolution. Agriculture is thus derivative, but since it has led to a disequilibrium between man and the environment it is difficult to judge it as an advance.

It has been estimated that a hunter and a gatherer needs about 20 km^2 to sustain himself and yet the same area under cultivation can support about 6000 people (Schwanitz, 1966). These figures should not be taken too seriously, but they do indicate the possibilities for population growth that have faced man since the beginnings of agriculture. The present size and rate of increase of the population of tropical Africa can thus be attributed to the introduction of cultivated crops and a rapid improvement in the techniques of agriculture. This has happened mainly in the last thousand years or so, but especially in the last three or four hundred years since the arrival of the Europeans. The advanced techniques of agriculture now advocated should result in an even more spectacular increase in human numbers.

Crops are derived from wild species of plants, but in many cases the wild ancestor is no longer in existence. It is not clear why this should be so but possibly the wild species could not counter the competition from the cultivated forms. Almost all of the many plants now cultivated were discovered and developed a long time ago, in many cases thousands of years ago. One of the curiosities of the discovery of the mechanism of heredity just over a hundred years ago and the subsequent development of the science of genetics is that no new crop of major importance has come to light, unless we include a species of dandelion grown in Russia and the development of cultivated varieties of blueberry in North America. It appears that virtually all the possible plants had been tried by the earlier cultivators and modern genetics has merely been able to improve existing species of crops. The genetic improvement of crops has been done most competently and there are now thousands of varieties of some crops, such as rice, each of them suitable for cultivation in a rather narrow range of ecological conditions. Many cultivated plants are hybrids and some are polyploids. Their genetics is in many cases well understood and every year new and improved varieties of one crop or another are being marketed. Until recently, improvement simply meant increasing the yield, but now increasing effort is being devoted to the improvement of the nutritional value of certain crops, particularly of traditional staples that have a low protein content.

Most of the crops now grown for food or for cash in tropical Africa come either from south-east Asia or South America. The savanna regions of Africa have provided a few food crops, notably sorghum, but the forest has contributed little. There seems to be no obvious explanation for this, except that there was little or no early experimentation with wild plants in the forest region. If this is so there should be some potential food crops in the African forests. But more probably the paucity of plant species of the African forests compared with those of South America and south-east Asia provides the clue. Whatever the reason the human population in the forest region of Africa is now dependent mainly on food crops introduced from elsewhere.

It was the custom of the Portuguese explorers of the fifteenth, sixteenth, and seventeenth centuries to carry with them in their boats the seeds of plants that might prove useful should they set foot on land where the seeds could be planted and the crops grown. There is evidence that many of the early introductions of crops into tropical Africa were made by the Portuguese, and once introduced the crops spread overland so that later European explorers were sometimes astonished to find crops of obvious outside origin growing in areas where no white man had been before. Some crops were repeatedly introduced, many being introduced independently into East and into West Africa. The early history of these introductions can be traced by studying the local name of the crop in different languages and by its appearance in recognizable form as ornamentation on earthenware containers. In addition there are written records kept by the early explorers in the form of log books and diaries. Translations of early Portuguese manuscripts are providing particularly good records of the early introductions of crops into Africa. It is however a pity that there is not more collaboration between historians and biologists as some of the translations into English refer to plants (and animals) that in all probability have never occurred in tropical Africa.

The history of the introduction of maize into tropical Africa provides a good example of the way in which historical and biological research can be combined in order to trace the spread of a crop over a large area in a short time. Maize is the most distinctive of all crops and it is placed in a separate genus from all other grasses. It originated in tropical America, probably as a hybrid between two wild species of grass. As a crop its chief advantage lies in the enormous size of the seeds which are far bigger than those produced by other grasses that have been developed as crops. It has been cultivated in South and Central America for thousands of years and is particularly amenable to selective breeding and hybridization. It cannot propagate itself and the seeds have to be released from the cob before they can germinate. Its existence is thus entirely dependent upon cultivation, and hence wherever it appears it must have been introduced by man, unlike many of the grain crops which are able to seed themselves and grow wild. Soon after the discovery of America by Columbus maize was spread rapidly to many parts of the world and in some areas it became a major food crop. Today it is the third most important crop in tropical Africa, most of it being grown by cultivators to feed their own families, although in some areas, notably Kenya, maize marketing boards have been set up and a considerable trade is developing.

There are two opinions as to how and when maize first entered Africa: one that it was introduced after the discovery of America by Columbus, and the other that it occurred in Africa before that date. A third possibility, that it was independently developed in Africa as a crop, is not seriously entertained. The first view is discussed by Miracle (1966). On the basis of linguistic evidence he suggests that maize penetrated into the interior of Africa from both the west and the east coast, possibly having been first introduced by the Portuguese, who, it is believed, were motivated to grow the crop as a means of supplying cheap food for their slaves. It is also possible that maize arrived from the north with the Arab traders, but the date of its first occurrence in the northern savanna is not known. The crop appears to have spread rather slowly from the coastal regions and it may not have reached Uganda (where it is now an important food) until about 1861. The second view is propounded by Jeffreys (1967), with special reference to the occurrence of maize in southern Africa. Jeffreys points out that when Vasco da Gama reached Mozambique in 1498 he found maize already present and cites many other sources of evidence, some linguistic and some based on Portuguese records, that suggest that maize occurred in southern Africa before the arrival of Columbus in America in 1492. The Portuguese word for maize is *milho* and Jeffreys says that they used the word *milhom* for maize as long ago as 1289, over two hundred years before Columbus reached America.[1] If Jeffreys is right the question arises as to how maize first reached Africa, and indeed how it spread from America in pre-Columbian times. Jeffreys suggests that the crop was first introduced into the eastern coastal region by the Arabs and cites early tribal names for the crop as evidence of its occurrence before the time of Columbus. There is a school of thought that advocates that there was contact between Africa and South America before the time of Columbus. The idea has never been substantiated, but if there was contact this would immediately explain the early arrival of maize in Africa, as undoubtedly the seeds would be an obvious part of the cargo of any vessel venturing from South America to Africa.

[1] It is possible that the Portuguese confused maize with sorghum.

Historians and anthropologists are hesitant to admit the possibility of human contact between South America and Africa before the time of Columbus. It seems to me, however, that some contact is extremely likely. An analogous situation exists in the butterfly fauna of Madagascar, most of which must have originated in Africa and colonized Madagascar through chance dispersal across the sea which at its narrowest point is 400 km wide. Butterflies can of course fly but the distance is too great for more than the occasional arrival, but given time it is likely that a considerable number of individuals made the journey safely and established populations. Why then should not the occasional vessel carrying people cross the southern Atlantic safely? There has been plenty of time for such an event to have occurred.

But despite the above considerations maize did not become an important crop in Africa until the present century. Its early cultivation seems to be associated with the need for travellers to provide cheap food for slaves and bearers but exactly how the crop first got to Africa remains a mystery.

The early history of the introduction of most other crops contains a similar amount of ambiguity. The initial introductions seem to have occurred on the coast and at first the crops spread rather slowly into the interior, the rate of spread rapidly gaining momentum as time passed. Some crops appear to have been brought across the Sahara by people from the north. The mode of dispersal seems to have been dictated by the necessity to carry seeds and to plant and grow them wherever suitable land was found and whenever there was sufficient time.

The environment of tropical Africa is diverse and there is a complex mosaic of land, some fertile and some barren, but each area more or less suitable or unsuitable for some of the enormous variety of tropical crops that are now available. Cultivation must have proceeded by a series of trials and errors, in which years of famine and plenty occurred with conspicuous unpredictability. In this way a selective process operated, but no one knows how many people perished or were forced to migrate and become integrated with other groups as crop after crop failed. Entire ethnic groups may have been exterminated during the trial and error period of cultivation. It is possible to envisage the gradual transfer of skills and knowledge acquired by hunting and gathering to cultivating and the raising of livestock. Groups of people that succeeded expanded in numbers until they themselves either had to move or perish. Knowledge acquired was transmitted verbally from generation to generation so that eventually many cultivators became expert in their own environment; but transferred to a slightly different environment their knowledge might prove totally inadequate. The failure of the notorious ground-nut scheme in what was Tanganyika is an excellent example of such a situation in which despite the technical knowledge of the European agriculturalists there was insufficient understanding of the ecology of the region, resulting in enormous financial loss, and, it may be added, some loss of prestige.

A cultivator who has grown up in an area where traditions have been passed from one generation to the next can accurately judge by looking at the natural vegetation the suitability of a piece of land for the cultivation of a specific crop. He will probably have acquired a vocabulary of hundreds of names for plants, trees, and vegetation associations, and will be fully aware of the significance of what might be called indicator plants when planning his activities (Allan, 1965). His knowledge, if it could be formulated properly, would delight even theoretical ecologists; indeed the experienced cultivator is an expert ecologist in his own environment, but when displaced from it he may well face disaster. This knowledge has been developed in response to pressures exerted by the environment and without it survival would be even more hazardous.

Shifting cultivation was presumably evolved as a natural response to successive changes in the quality of the land as cultivation of the same area brought about reductions in the productivity of the crop. The phenomenon cannot be explained in any other way, although there may be in addition complex ritual beliefs involved in changing the centre of operations from one place to another. Thus there are, all through Africa, small areas of apparently fertile land that have never been cultivated, or at least not cultivated for a very long time. These areas usually turn out to be sacred or perhaps are dedicated to the spirits, and they may remain uncultivated even in times of famine. Allan (1965) describes a piece of fertile land in West Africa that had remained uncultivated through fear of a powerful spirit. A group of young men, recent converts to Christianity, returned to the nearby village and asked the chief if they might use the land for growing vegetables. This was opposed by the villagers, but the case was referred to the chief's court which gave the following judgement: 'Let these ridiculous young men have their garden. If they die, it will not be our fault, for we have done our best to dissuade them. If they do not die, it will only show that we have been mistaken in supposing that this is a sacred place.'

The evolution of land tenure, an extremely complex subject in Africa, can possibly be traced from the hunting and gathering territories of former times. There is much ritual and politics involved in who has rights in land and who may be allowed to cultivate it. But the result of this is that in one way or another the available land is apportioned out among the people, each family group receiving and holding with variable rights an amount of land that is considered appropriate to its needs. Disputes over land, although frequent, are not as common as might be expected, and there is considerable understanding as to who has rights over an area and the extent to which these rights can be interpreted. The sharing of land among the members of a group (such as a village) is analogous to the way in which animals like birds share out a space into territories: some individuals because of their status relative to others, receive better shares than others, and there is rarely direct conflict over who has rights in an area.

In the past few years detailed monographs have been prepared on the botany and cultivation of tropical crops. Many of the more important species have now been dealt with and much is known about how and where they can be most effectively grown. In tropical Africa crops are grown in a way that is not especially productive, mainly because each family tends to grow just enough for its own consumption. Governments and private enterprises have in recent years started programmes of growing and marketing certain crops on a larger and, they hope, more efficient scale. There are many problems associated with growing tropical crops, not the least of which is the extraordinary complexity of insect damage and the transmission of disease, which together create ecological predicaments whose magnitude is unparalleled in temperate regions. The overriding importance of insects in agriculture is discussed in the next chapter, but I first want to discuss the biology of some of the more common

5 Roots of cassava. This crop, introduced from tropical America, is easily grown and is relatively free from pests and diseases, but it contains virtually no protein.

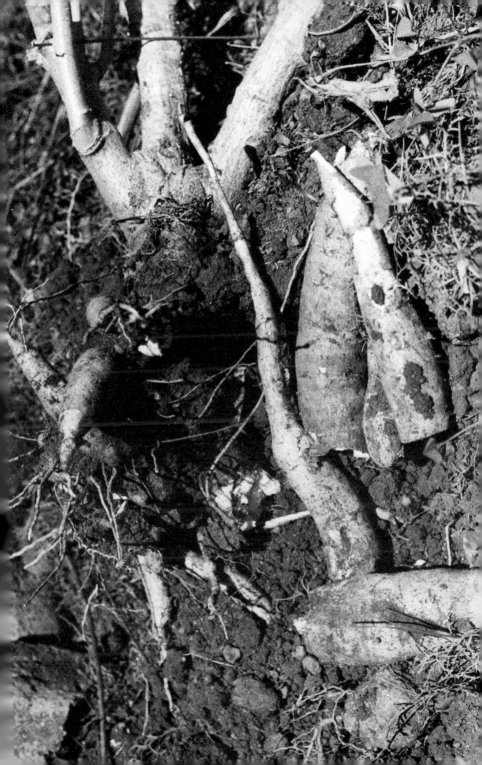

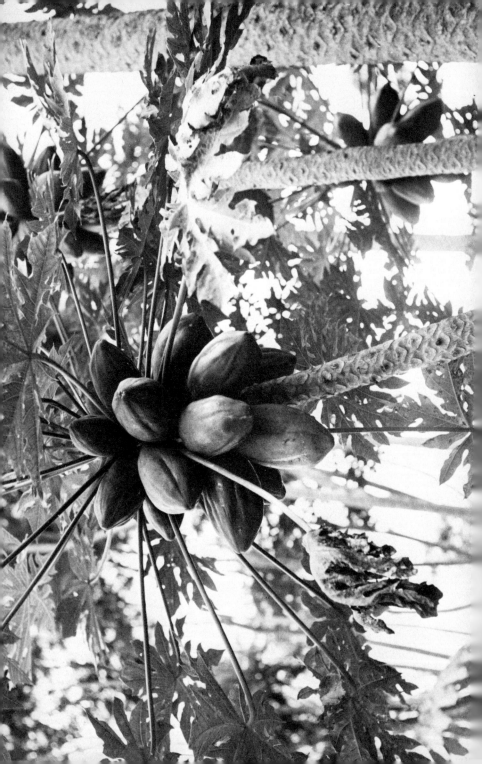

plants used as crops in tropical Africa, some of the information being derived from Cobley (1956) and Purseglove (1968) who have provided an introduction to the biology of tropical crops.

All the cereal crops are derived from grasses of the family Gramineae. Most of them are represented by a single species with an immense number of varieties that have been selectively bred by man. As grasses are rare in tropical forest it would appear that most of the cereal crops are derived from savanna and grassy environments, and indeed many grow best where the rainfall is not excessive, while some cannot tolerate high temperatures. The important species now grown in tropical Africa are rice, *Oryza sativa*, sorghum, *Sorghum vulgare*, maize, *Zea mays*, bulrush millet, *Pennisetum typhoideum*, panicum millet, *Panicum* spp., finger millet, *Eleusine coracana*, and hungry rice, *Digitaria exilis*.

In West Africa in particular, rice is rapidly becoming the favourite cereal food and the amount of land devoted to its cultivation is increasing rapidly every year. There are thousands of different varieties of rice that differ genetically, morphologically, and physiologically from each other. The crop thrives in the wetter tropics and is usually planted in natural or irrigated swamps. In West Africa, the young rice plants are planted by hand in the swamps soon after the onset of the wet season, the land having first been cleared of weeds, and in areas where irrigation is possible, the soil is first flooded. The plant grows in standing water and is harvested early in the dry season. In many areas only one crop is produced a year, although it is perfectly possible to produce two crops provided planting and harvesting are performed quickly and without delays. It is common practice to grow other crops on the same land in the dry season once the water level has subsided. Mangrove swamps are being reclaimed on a large scale in West Africa and are being developed as rice fields. Swamp rice fields provide an ideal environment for the species of snails that are intermediate hosts for schistosomiasis and many of the people who plant and harvest rice suffer from this disease. The rice fields also encourage the growth of mosquito populations which transmit malaria and other diseases. Several varieties of upland rice are also cultivated. Upland rice does not require standing water and it is usually grown on hillsides in high rainfall areas in the wet season. The land is first cleared of bush (or

6 Fruits of pawpaw. This crop was introduced into Africa from tropical America. It is quick to colonize abandoned farmland and now occurs in a semi-wild state.

forest) by slashing and burning, and the crop planted out on the steep slopes of the hill. The same area is used for only one or two seasons as the quality of the soil rapidly deteriorates through erosion and loss of nutrients. The cultivation of upland rice is thus usually a destructive process and is unlikely to continue indefinitely as land becomes more valuable and scarce.

Sorghum is a tall grass, the grains of which form a major item of diet for people living in the savanna. There are many varieties, some of local distribution, and each adapted to a rather narrow range of conditions. Some varieties are more or less drought resistant, an important consideration in the drier savanna where rainfall is sparse and unpredictable. Sorghum is evidently derived from a wild African grass and hence it was one of the first crops to be cultivated in Africa.

Maize grows better in rather damper situations than sorghum, but varieties that are relatively drought resistant have been bred, and these are being introduced into savanna areas. Some varieties of maize grow to a height of three to five metres, but in tropical Africa the crop is usually heavily infested with the larvae of stem-boring moths and most of the plants seen are much smaller than this. Maize is often planted interspersed with other crops, but there is an attempt to encourage large-scale production. The possibility of breeding varieties that contain a higher proportion of protein is being investigated.

The word millet is used to describe several distinct species of grasses that produce small grains. They are grown mainly for local consumption along with other grains, and there has been no attempt at large-scale marketing. The bulrush or pearl millet is thought to have originated in the grasslands of central Africa, and it is now grown throughout the savanna areas cultivated with sorghum, doing better than sorghum on sandy and light soils. It is grown in the wet season and produces a crop very quickly, and is thus a useful standby if food is short. Several species of *Panicum* (a large genus) are cultivated in a similar way, and in general they can survive better under hot and dry conditions than maize or sorghum, which most people prefer because of their high yields. Finger millet is another local species, cultivated especially in damper areas, and used chiefly when other sources of grain are in short supply.

Hungry rice, as the name implies, is grown and used when rice is scarce. The plant is unknown in the wild state and yet it requires little attention during cultivation. It is a staple crop among people living in the drier savanna areas of West Africa.

The sugar cane, *Saccharum officinarum*, is also a member of the grass family, apparently originating in tropical Asia although its wild ancestor is not known. The plant is unusual in that its metabolic processes lead to the storage of sugar rather than other carbohydrates, but not until quite recently were its potentialities fully realized as a major source of sugar. Before the use of cane sugar (and later sugar beet) sweetening was a matter of adding honey or the secretions of trees to food or drink. Sugar is grown mainly as a cash crop in plantations in areas of moderate or high rainfall. Its cultivation requires a great deal of manpower as the stems are bulky and difficult to transport. Most of the crop is processed and packaged, but people also chew the stems and suck out the sweet juice. Many varieties of sugar cane have been bred, some of them polyploids which produce plants with varying quantities of sugar in the stems, but able to grow under an increasingly wide variety of ecological conditions. In East Africa considerable quantities are produced, some of it being processed in the distillation of alcohol for commercial use. Most of the packaged sugar sold in Africa is imported, and even in small villages it is possible to buy packets of sugar imported from Britain, China, and other countries.

Peas and beans, often collectively known as pulses, are the seeds of a variety of plants in the family Papilionaceae. Plants in this family develop nodules in their roots through a symbiotic association with certain bacteria which convert atmospheric nitrogen into nitrates. Not only are the plants an important source of protein for food, but they also enrich soil that is deficient in nitrogen. Throughout the world pulse crops are alternated with other crops so as to replenish the soil with nitrogen. Many of the cultivated beans originated in the New World tropics and until recently selective breeding of most of the species has been localized and on a small scale. In areas of tropical Africa where meat and fish are scarce, peas and beans probably form the main source of protein in the diet of the people. But despite this the growing of pulses has not been developed in Africa to the extent that it has in tropical America where almost every dish contains beans in one form or another. Many of the important crop species belong to the genus *Phaseolus* in Africa and they are usually grown mixed with cereal and root crops. The cow-pea, *Vigna unguiculata*, is one of the few species that seems to have originated in Africa, and it is widely cultivated in humid regions. The ground-nut (or peanut), *Arachis hypogaea*, is becoming increasingly important as a cash crop from which vegetable oil is derived. It is now grown on plantations in many African countries, and it is important in the diet of people in West and Central Africa. It would appear that the problem of protein malnutrition could be largely solved if people could be persuaded to grow and eat more beans and ground-nuts.

People in the humid areas of Africa depend heavily on starchy root crops as their most important source of food. Most of the root crops are grown on a small scale, but they occur everywhere, replacing the grain crops of the savanna. They seem to suffer less from insect damage than the grain crops and, being easy to cultivate, they provide a ready source of food for the expanding populations in the forest region. All are poor in protein content, and the widespread occurrence of malnutrition in the humid tropics can be largely attributed to the dependence of the people on root crops. Sweet potato, *Ipomoea batatas*, a member of the Convolvulaceae, originated in South America, and is now grown throughout Africa wherever the rainfall is sufficiently high. The genus *Ipomoea* contains about four hundred tropical species and it is remarkable that only one of them has produced a useful crop. Cassava, *Manihot esculenta*, also from South America, is possibly the easiest of all crops to grow. It is remarkably free from pests and diseases and can be grown by simply planting the cut stems in shallow soil. The ease with which it is grown undoubtedly accounts for its widespread use, and it is a pity that the roots contain almost no protein. Like some of the millets it is often used as a famine relief crop. In terms of nutritional value it probably qualifies as the worst food in the world. Cassava is a member of the Euphorbiaceae and the genus *Manihot* contains over 150 species, but none except the cultivated species is of economic importance.

Yams, *Dioscorea* spp., belong to a family of climbing monocotyledons, the Dioscoreaceae, which are related to the lilies. They form

an important staple crop in West Africa. Like cassava the plants
and the tubers are relatively free from insect pests and, being easy
to cultivate, they are grown everywhere in and around towns and
villages. There are about six species, apparently originating in the
tropics of south-east Asia and the Pacific, and they quickly spread
into Africa as contact with the rest of the world was established. The
coco-yam, *Colocasia antiquorum*, a member of the Araceae, apparently originated in eastern Asia or the Pacific, and is now widely
cultivated in West African village gardens. The edible portion, the
corm, contains more protein than is present in other root crops, and
also contains substantial amounts of vitamins.

One of the most remarkable achievements of agriculture has been
the transformation of the small, seed-producing, and inedible wild
banana into an enormous and complex variety of large, seedless, and
edible fruits. The genetics and evolution of bananas has been discussed in detail by Simmonds (1962). Bananas, *Musa* spp., belong
to the Musaceae, a family of plants found in the wild in Africa and
tropical Asia. All the edible varieties are derived from plants indigenous to south-east Asia. Bananas are commercial crops in the
West Indies and the Canary Islands; there has been some development of an export trade in West Africa, mainly in the Ivory Coast,
but in most of Africa they are grown for local consumption. There
are two main uses of bananas, some varieties being used as fruits
and others (the plantains) cooked as vegetables. They grow well in
the more humid parts of Africa, even fairly high up on mountains
where it is cool, and are relatively free from pests and diseases.

Citrus belongs to the Rutaceae, and probably originated in Asia;
it includes several species of edible fruits, including grapefruit, *C.
paradisi*, orange, *C. sinensis*, lemon, *C. limon*, lime, *C. aurantifolia*,
and tangerine, *C. reticulata*. All of these are cash crops in areas
outside tropical Africa, including South Africa, but in tropical
Africa they are grown in gardens and villages for local consumption.
The fruits are rich in vitamin C and they are extremely popular,
being conspicuous items in local markets. In West Africa most of
the fruit is produced towards the end of the dry season and at this
time the smell of citrus is one of the most striking features of some
of the West African cities, such as Accra and Freetown. Citrus trees
are heavily infested with insects and to grow the crop effectively

much attention has to be devoted to pest control. In West Africa little attention is paid to the effects of pests and the productivity of the trees is low, but since trees are allowed to grow almost anywhere this is not a serious problem.

The mango, *Mangifera indica*, a member of the Anacardiaceae, which rivals citrus in popularity, originated in tropical Asia. There is much variation in the quality of the fruit, and the best results are obtained by grafting. The seeds germinate well and in many parts of Africa the trees now grow in a semi-wild state, and indeed in parts of West Africa mango trees are among the more frequent colonizers of secondary forest. Pineapple, *Ananas comosa*, a member of the Bromeliaceae, originated in tropical America, and is now grown throughout Africa for local consumption and to a small extent as a plantation crop. It is propagated vegetatively, and is drought resistant, so is an important fruit in low rainfall areas. The pawpaw, *Carica papaya*, a member of the Caricaceae, is also from tropical America. It grows well from seeds and occurs around houses in almost all villages. The male and female plants are separate individuals and it is the custom to cut all but a few of the males down within a limited area and to leave the females growing. Numerous other fruits are grown in gardens, many of them being allowed to germinate anywhere. Among these are the guava, *Psidium guajava*, a member of the Myrtaceae, and various species of *Anona*, belonging to the Anonaceae, which are common around villages, but are rarely specifically cultivated. Almost all the fruits grown in tropical Africa are introduced from tropical America or from south-east Asia. There are plenty of fruits available, the different kinds tending to succeed each other as the seasons change. Most are eaten whole and uncooked and they are probably an important source of vitamins.

An enormous variety of vegetables is grown in the villages. Most are produced for local consumption, and although local markets handle considerable quantities, there is effectively no export of vegetable crops. In dry areas species of Cucurbitaceae are of paramount importance. Most of the species, including marrow, cucumber, and the numerous varieties of gourds, originated in tropical America and south-east Asia, but the water melon is African. In some areas they are used as a source of water in the dry season and some varieties are used as containers for liquids. The family Solanaceae also contains a variety of vegetable crops, including the egg-plant or aubergine, *Solanum melongena*, a native of India, now grown in many areas of Africa, and various forms of tomato, *Lycopersicon esculentum*, a native of Central and South America, and in Africa much in demand for sauces. Okra, *Hibiscus esculentus*, a member of the Malvaceae, originated in Central Africa, and is grown extensively as a vegetable, both the fruit and the leaves being used. Avocado, *Persea americana*, a member of the Lauraceae, originated in Central America and is now common throughout tropical Africa. It is of considerable nutritional value because the fruits contain much oil and protein. The bread-fruit and the jack-fruit, *Artocarpus communis* and *A. integra*, members of the Moraceae, are related to figs and originated in south-east Asia. They grow in a semi-wild state in many parts of West Africa, but they can hardly be described as popular items of food.

Many of the vegetable crops grown in temperate areas will also produce well in certain areas of tropical Africa. Thus cabbages, lettuces, onions, and so on, grow in gardens almost anywhere, but they cannot be said to be important crops, functioning chiefly as additions to the staples. There are also a number of plants that are in Sierra Leone referred to as 'greens'. These include species that plantation growers might regard as weeds, but around villages they are encouraged to grow and are collected for use in sauces and as flavouring. One of the most popular in the Freetown area is *Portulaca* sp., a common weed of rice fields. It produces pleasant-tasting leaves at the beginning of the rains and grows well on soil that has recently been prepared for cultivation.

The three important world beverages, tea, coffee, and cocoa, are all tropical. All three are an important source of outside money in several African countries. Tea, *Camellia sinensis*, belongs to the Theaceae, and is grown commercially in East Africa on hilly acid soils with rather a high rainfall. Most of that grown is exported, and some is re-imported after being blended and packaged. Tea is a popular drink throughout tropical Africa. The plant and its many varieties originated in Asia and it requires a considerable amount of attention if a good crop is to be produced. Coffee, *Coffea arabica*, a member of the Rubiaceae, originated in Ethiopia, and with

C. canephora, originally from the Congo, and *C. liberica*, from West
Africa, is a crop of great importance to the economy of many African
countries. Large quantities are grown on plantations, but much is
also grown by small farmers and sold to marketing boards. It is
rather an easy crop to grow, but good quality coffee requires much
attention. It has been necessary to restrict the amount of coffee
grown in some countries in order to avoid a world surplus and hence
a fall in prices. Cocoa, *Theobroma cacao*, a member of the Sterculiaceae, originated from South America and is now grown extensively
as a forest crop in West Africa, especially in Nigeria, the Ivory
Coast, Cameroon, and Ghana, where the export of cocoa provides
an important source of income.

Cotton, *Gossypium* spp., belonging to the Malvaceae, is the most
important fibre crop in the world, and in Africa it is grown in drier
areas on rather large plantations, but also by peasant farmers. The
numerous species and varieties of cotton have apparently originated
from plants that occur in all the major tropical regions of the
world. Sisal, *Agave* spp., belonging to the Agavaceae, is an important
source of fibre and plantations have been developed along the East
African coast. The crop originated in Central and South America.
The future of sisal and cotton in world trade is uncertain as more
and more synthetic fibres are produced and the demand for natural
products decreases. There are many other fibre-producing plants
grown in tropical Africa, mostly on a small scale and for local use,
and there is enormous opportunism in the use of wild plants as a
source of fibre for basket making and other purposes.

Some fruits are utilized as a source of vegetable oils. In tropical
Africa the most important species are the ground-nut, the castor oil
plant, *Ricinus communis*, a member of the Euphorbiaceae, the coconut, *Cocos nucifera*, and the oil palm, *Elaeis guineensis*, both Palmae.
The oil palm is a native of West Africa and huge plantations have
been developed in some areas as there is much demand for the oil
on the world market. This crop, together with sorghum and coffee,
is one of the few native African plants that has been extensively
introduced to other tropical regions of the world.

Numerous spices and drugs are cultivated, mostly on a small
scale for local use. The most important commercial crop is tobacco,
Nicotiana tabacum, a member of the Solanaceae. The smoking of

tobacco is widespread and most countries now manufacture their own cigarettes, the tobacco being in many cases imported from elsewhere. The cultivation of pyrethrum, *Pyrethrum cinerariaefolium*, a member of the Compositae, as a source of insecticide, seems likely to develop into a major industry in East Africa, especially now that the dangers of synthetic insecticides are more fully appreciated. Pyrethrum, like many other plants contains repellent substances in its tissues which can be extracted and processed as an effective insecticide that is less dangerous to human health than such insecticides as DDT.

The bulk of the crops grown in Africa are consumed by the people that plant them. Many are marketed locally, but only a relatively small number, the most important being tea, coffee, cocoa, cotton, and the fruits producing vegetable oils, reach the international markets.

There is as much variation in the ways crops are grown as there is in the crops themselves, and generalization is difficult. I shall therefore describe the seasonal cycle of events in the cultivation of one small patch of land in Sierra Leone that I have observed for three successive years.

The main crop produced in this area is swamp rice, and all other activities are centred around the cultivation of this crop which is the only one that can be sold. It is convenient to start at the onset of the rainy season in June when the fields that are to be irrigated are cleared by hand of the weeds and the remains of the crops that have been grown during the dry season. First the weeds and other vegetation are cut down and then the land turned over, not deeply, and levelled. As the rains develop the fields begin to flood and irrigation channels are opened. The rice seedlings are planted by hand in July in the now flooded fields. Weeds grow rapidly and some attempt is made to control them, but they frequently overtake the efforts of the cultivators. The work is difficult in the torrential rain and the heat and humidity do not encourage the expenditure of too much effort. The rice grows throughout the wet season, reaching its full height in November and producing seeds in December. As the seeds ripen hordes of weaver birds come to feed on them, and small boys armed with slings are employed to drive the birds away. At times various juju symbols are erected either to discourage pests or to stop possible stealing of the crop by other people. The fact that stealing hardly ever occurs confirms the efficacy of the jujus. The rice is harvested by hand in December and the fields begin to dry up. By about February the land is turned over again and a little later a wide variety of plants is grown. These include maize, water melon, ground-nuts, beans of various kinds, sweet potatoes, and cassava, the latter being grown especially around the edges of the irrigated fields. The crops are grown mixed together so that even within a few square metres one can see four or five different species growing. Peppers, egg-plant, and okra are grown on the more upland areas surrounding the rice fields. Harvesting of these crops takes place in a somewhat haphazard way throughout the dry season, but the impression is that only what is required for immediate local consumption is gathered. This means that in some dry seasons the bulk of what is produced is abandoned. I have seen water melons rotting in hundreds, mainly because there were too many and there was no ready market in which they could be sold. By the end of the dry season both planting and harvesting have stopped and the land becomes overgrown with weeds and re-mains like this until the rain commences and preparations are made for the next crop of rice.

All the crops suffer from the attacks of insect pests. The larvae of stem-boring flies, Diopsidae, bore into the rice stems, but no attempt is made to control these insects. This would in any case be difficult without the application of insecticides. Maize grows well at first, but later begins to suffer from the larvae of stem-boring moths, and then as the grains ripen they are attacked and destroyed by *Zonocerus variegatus*, a large, slow-moving grasshopper, which could easily be removed and destroyed by hand, but which is ignored. In most years the bulk of the maize crop is destroyed by these grasshoppers but no one seems alarmed. Almost all the pods of beans are bored into by the larvae of butterflies of the family Lycaenidae, and again no attempt is made to control these pests. Indeed it is remarkable that considering the effort devoted to scaring off birds and putting up juju symbols so little attention is paid to insect damage. It is almost as if the people do not see the insects. Once I found that a man had planted out some orange seeds the new cotyledons of which were just appearing. On almost every plant there was a larva of the butterfly, *Papilio demodocus*, which would rapidly grow so large that it would destroy the tiny plant. When I pointed this out to the man he said that he would try to find someone to pick off the larvae, but he was in no hurry, and although he seemed to appreciate my interest in his crop, he was not concerned about the damage the larvae were causing.

In this area, as in many others, food can be grown in abundance, and losses from pests are taken for granted. It is only in the drier areas where food may be seasonally scarce that the people take a serious interest in the damage caused by pests and take preventive measures by removing the insects from their crops. There is little doubt that the productivity of this part of Sierra Leone is only a fraction of what it could be. I do not necessarily feel that this attitude is to be deplored. Indeed the attitude has much to commend it, for why take the trouble to improve the crops when enough can be grown with relatively little effort? The large variety of crops grown, especially in the dry season, ensures that failures of one or more crops are not of great consequence: there are always some crops that do well enough to feed the people. Rice, however, is taken seriously, chiefly because it can be sold, but it is perhaps strange that an effort to grow more than one crop of rice a year is not made.

It is easy to be critical of the efforts to grow crops in rural Africa but it is also possible that farmers in developed countries, with their highly mechanized methods, pesticides, weed-killers, and fertilizers, have something to learn from the peasant farmers of Africa. Thus it now appears that under certain circumstances the yield of cabbages in Britain can be increased if some weeds are allowed to grow with the crop. This is because the weeds provide a habitat for a diversity of predators (insects and spiders) that feed on the pests of the cabbages. Without the weeds there are fewer predators and cabbages suffer more from pests. African peasant farmers do not in general make special efforts to eradicate weeds and it is possible they have discovered, through trial and error, that by leaving many of the weeds alone the yield of the crop is increased. It is equally possible that the custom of growing a variety of crops in a small area decreases the risk of the destruction of the crops by pests as a diversity of crops is likely to result in a greater spectrum of useful predators of pests.

There are flourishing markets in most of the towns and many of the villages that sell agricultural products from the rural areas. It would seem that these markets are playing an increasingly important part in the economy of the people, but the money that changes hands contributes little to the economy of the country as a whole, as there is little possibility of taxation. Most of the products sold are uncooked fruits and vegetables, and the markets resemble those found in similar situations in Europe.

The financial state of a nation is largely dependent on the nature and volume of its exports to other countries. Africa exports raw materials, especially plant products and minerals. The chief characteristic of the export trade of African countries is the supreme importance of one or two commodities. There is little diversification and so each nation relies upon a crop that happens to grow well or on a mineral that happens to occur in abundance. About three-quarters of the exports from Ghana are of unprocessed cocoa. The Gambia depends almost entirely on the export of ground-nuts, while Liberia is dependent on rubber. Other countries are in a similar position, several of them being heavily dependent on the uncertain world market for coffee. It is however only in the last fifty years that cash crops have become important in the economy of countries in tropical Africa. Thus in about 1909 cotton first began to be exported from Uganda, but the rate of production rose almost geometrically so that by about 1960 Uganda was exporting about 400 thousand bales, each weighing about 140 kg, and had become a major producer of this commodity. A similar trend occurred in the Congo, developing about ten years later than in Uganda. Again, in Uganda the growing and marketing of coffee has been particularly productive in recent years. Most of the coffee is grown by small farmers, and with the demand for raw materials for the manufacture of instant coffee, the quality of the berries has not been a major consideration. Coffee production in Uganda quadrupled between 1949 and 1959, and the crop is now of considerable importance in the national economy.

Research on tropical crops is aimed directly or indirectly at improving productivity. This may be achieved in a variety of ways: breeding varieties of the crop that are better adapted to local conditions, finding ways of reducing the destructive effects of insects and other pests, and improving the quality and marketing facilities of fertilizers which if applied should raise the yield. Many national and some international organizations exist solely for these purposes. The problem of dependence on a single plant commodity as an export is that there is the danger that the depredations of an insect or a disease may in quite a short time almost completely ruin the harvest, and hence the economy of the country. This has happened in the past, and as more and more land is subjected to the cultivation of single crops it can be expected to be an increasing economic hazard. It is thus possible that a population adapted to the growing of crops for its own needs is better adapted to the environment than one that aims to increase its export of a single plant product. Natural communities comprising a diversity of species tend to be more stable than those containing few species. I do not want to carry this analogy too far but it seems to me that if, as we are told, the future of Africa lies in improving the agriculture, then it would seem desirable that some of this improvement should be directed towards diversification.

CHAPTER 6

Weeds, Pests, and Diseases of Cultivation

Weeds are plants that grow wherever man cultivates the soil and which in one way or another reduce the quantity and sometimes the quality of the crop. From this it follows that where there is no cultivation there are no weeds. Many species that have become weeds have a considerable capacity for vegetative reproduction and an ability to withstand extreme changes in the environment. Some species have a considerable genetic potential and can quickly evolve genotypes that are well suited for changes in the environment brought about by man's activities. These evolutionary adaptations frequently involve the development of polyploids and the formation of what are called local ecotypes which, through the process of natural selection, ensure a rapid adjustment to changing circumstances. Some species of weeds respond very quickly indeed to a new environment, and it thus appears that weeds share many of the characteristics of the species of plants used as crops. In many areas of the world the most common and troublesome weeds are species introduced from elsewhere, but in the tropics most of the common agricultural weeds are members of the local flora that have exploited the special ecological conditions created by agriculture.

Pests are animals that reduce the productivity of crops. They share many of the biological features of weeds, but their ecological role is different. Weeds compete with crops for energy and nutrients and so lower the yield of the crop, whereas pests damage the crop either by consuming it or by transmitting diseases, especially virus and fungal diseases, which substantially lower the plant's capacity to survive. Pests are known from all the major groups of animals, but by far the most important are the insects. About four-fifths of the species of terrestrial animals are insects and with few exceptions almost all the major pests of cultivation are insects.

It is possible that nearly half the potential food production of tropical Africa is lost through the action of weeds and pests, and much effort has been and is being devoted to reducing this loss. The productivity of African agriculture is about the lowest in the world, and although a major cause of this may be lack of mechanization, the effects of weeds and pests are considerable. It was stated at an Organization for African Unity meeting in Addis Ababa in May 1967 that about 30 per cent of the grain stored in Africa is lost during storage alone, mostly being eaten by insects and rodents, but also through fungus diseases and, it was admitted, through bad handling.

The major weeds and pests of tropical Africa belong to native species that have exploited the cultivation of the land. A few species have been accidentally or deliberately introduced from other tropical areas of the world, but these are chiefly weeds and species of insects associated with grain crops. The role of insects as hazards to agriculture in Africa has been outlined by Uvarov (1961a, 1964) who points out that any tendency towards monocultures is likely to generate an increase in the population size of insects that feed on the crop or on related wild species. Uvarov mentions the introduction of large-scale mechanization in the cultivation of sorghum in the Sudan which resulted in heavy losses from local species of grasshoppers that had not previously been suspected as pests. Generally speaking it would appear that the diversity of species of crops grown by rural cultivators reduces to some extent the impact of insects on the crops, but any attempt to grow a crop on a large scale over a wide area encourages the build up of pest populations. It would therefore seem that plans to develop the agriculture by converting large areas of land to a single crop are doomed to failure unless precautions are taken to control the build-up of pest populations. These precautions must be ecologically oriented as it is often not known exactly which species will move in and devastate a crop. The conversion of much of the forest area of Africa to agriculture has resulted in an increase in grassland. Grasshoppers, which feed on grass, are rare in the forest, and thus by destroying the forest man has encouraged the spread and increase in abundance of grasshoppers. Cereal crops are grasses and since the cultivation of these tends to provide a better food supply for the grasshoppers than the wild grasses, damage from grasshoppers must continue to increase.

The effect of weeds and pests can be reduced by a variety of methods, not the least of which is the physical removal of the pest or weed from the crop by hand or by mechanical means. This works well for large and not too common species, but is highly uneconomical for smaller and more common species. There is also the problem of the availability and inclination of people to do the work. A commonly used method of ridding an area of pests and weeds is by the application of toxic chemicals. The action of these chemicals is to some extent selective so that only the undesirable species are affected, but there are other chemicals that destroy almost everything, harmful and harmless species. The danger of applying chemicals has been repeatedly emphasized in recent years, especially in relation to the ways in which chemicals can be picked up and concentrated in the food chain by other organisms, the end result being an increased risk to human consumers of crops. Both synthetic and natural chemicals are available. The natural chemicals make use of the toxic compounds present in plants which have evolved as a deterrent to herbivorous animals. The natural products seem less harmful to man and the environment than the synthetic chemicals.

Much interest has been generated by the possibility of biologically controlling weeds and pests. The basic concept of biological control is simple: animals that are known to feed selectively on weeds and pests are introduced into areas where the weeds and pests are a threat to the growing of a particular crop. This has sometimes produced spectacularly successful results. The possibility of controlling insect pests by genetic means is also being investigated. The most fruitful approach is to create strains of the insect pest in which one sex is infertile. These infertile individuals are then released into the pest population and although mating may take place there is a reduced production of offspring. Another possibility is the conversion of the pest population to all of one sex. Both of these approaches would seem to offer more hope than introducing predators and parasites which, because of the ways in which these are known to interact with their prey or hosts, are unlikely to do more than reduce the pest population temporarily. Another difficulty associated with introducing parasites and predators is that they may move on to other organisms that are harmless or indeed beneficial.

7 Fruits of mango. The mango was introduced from tropical Asia and, like the pawpaw, it now grows in a semi-wild state.

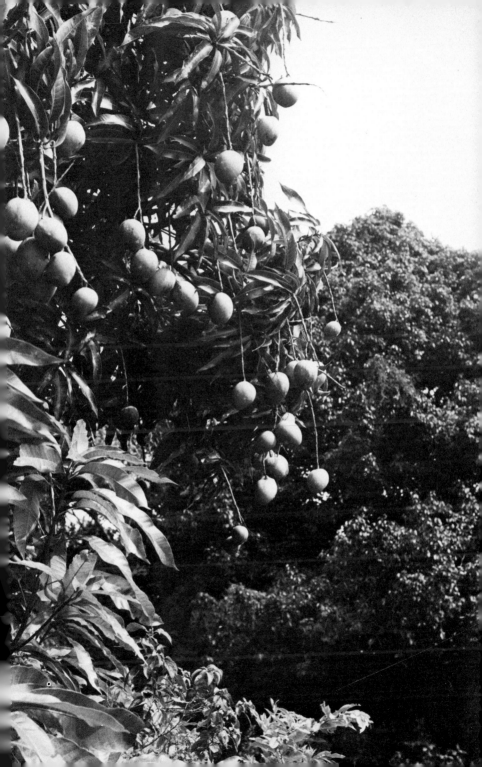

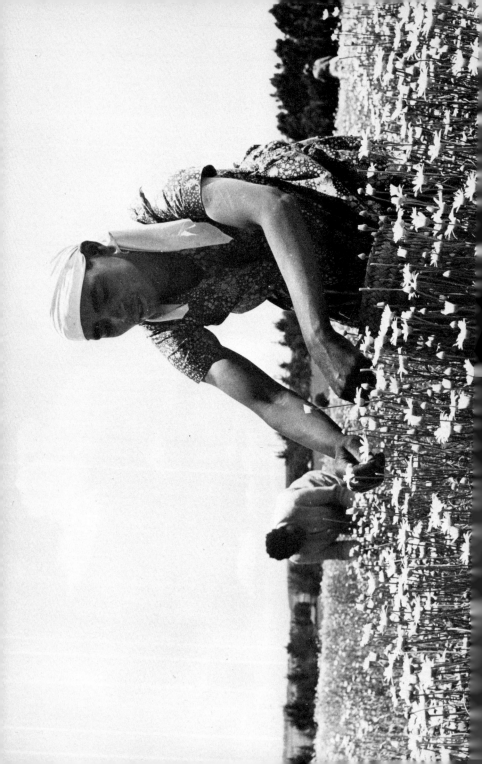

Throughout the world the roots of grain crops are attacked by a parasitic plant of the genus *Striga*. With the development of monocultures of grain crops, *Striga* tends to increase to such an extent that yields are reduced to almost nothing. In Northern Nigeria and in Kenya attempts have been made to use insects that attack *Striga* as a means of biologically controlling the parasite (Williams and Casswell, 1959; Davidson, 1963), but it is evident that if monocultures of grain crops continue to be encouraged in Africa a close watch will have to be kept on the spread of the parasite.

Lantana camara, a bushy member of the family Verbenaceae, is perhaps the most important and widespread weed in the tropics. It is a native of Central America, but has spread throughout the tropics, and in Africa occurs almost everywhere where man has disturbed the land. It forms dense thickets and grows rapidly tolerating both poor and dry soils, and can quickly colonize land that has been cleared for the growing of crops. It is remarkably resistant to slashing and burning, and its prickly texture and unpalatability to mammals make it difficult to eradicate. Apart from colonizing agricultural land, it also invades land that has been cleared of bush during attempts to control populations of tsetse flies, with the result that the flies quickly return to areas from which they have supposedly been eradicated. Indeed there is evidence that the spread of *Lantana* has extended the range of tsetse flies into areas of East Africa where previously they were absent (Greathead, 1968). On the credit side *Lantana* can colonize bare patches of ground that are subject to erosion, but the consensus is that the plant is a nuisance and should therefore be destroyed wherever possible. Much effort has been devoted to the possibility of controlling the spread of *Lantana* by introducing from elsewhere insects that feed on it. Entomologists who advise on programmes of biological control by this means are well aware of the numerous difficulties, the most important of which is to make sure that the introduced insect will not feed on other plants, especially on useful plants. *Teleonemia scrupulosa*, a lacebug of the family Tingidae has been used in attempts to control *Lantana*. The bug is a native of tropical America, and has been introduced into Hawaii, Fiji, Australia, Indonesia, India, Mauritius, and Africa in the hope that it will control *Lantana* (Davies and Greathead, 1967). In some areas there has been concern

8 Picking pyrethrum flowers in Kenya. The insecticide extracted from the flowers is extremely effective: it degrades in the presence of sunlight, and there is almost no insect resistance. Pyrethrum is thus from most points of view a better insecticide than DDT and similar compounds.

that the bug might move on to teak, a commercially important timber tree in the same family as *Lantana*, but teak seems relatively resistant to the attacks of insects because of the presence of a chemical repellent (Harley and Kunimoto, 1969). In Uganda *Teleonemia scrupulosa*, introduced to control *Lantana*, moved on to cultivated sesame, *Sesamum indicum*, which was totally unexpected as the plant is not related to *Lantana*; but survival of the bugs on the new host was poor and it was thought that there was little long-term danger (Davies and Greathead, 1967).

Like many weeds *Lantana* grows and reproduces rapidly and it is also genetically variable. The possibility arises, therefore, that if insects are repeatedly introduced to destroy it, resistant strains will evolve which cannot be eaten by insects. Many plants have evolved strains that are more or less resistant to the attacks of a wide spectrum of insects. In the case of *Lantana* a resistant strain would be favoured by natural selection and would spread rapidly through the population. The introduced insect would then either die out or move to another plant which could, of course, be a species of economic importance. This possibility is (or at least should be) a constant source of worry to those advocating biological control of weeds by introducing insects that feed on them. Indeed this method of biological control is unlikely to be completely effective except in special circumstances because as soon as the weed is decimated the insect population will be reduced in size, thus allowing for the possibility of the weed increasing again, and so on. In some instances where biological control of this sort has been implemented doubts have arisen as to whether the weed was controlled by the method used or by some other factors, and it has also been suggested that biological control discourages the cultivator from taking active steps to clear his land of weeds by other methods, such as by manual or mechanical weeding. The literature on the biological control of weeds has been extensively reviewed by Huffaker (1959) and Wilson (1964), both of whom raise considerable hopes that the method may prove to be increasingly successful, but also point out the difficulties that exist.

Two additional weeds have been introduced from tropical America and they both appear to be spreading rapidly throughout Africa wherever the land is disturbed by man. These two, *Tridax procum-*

bens, a member of the Compositae, and *Opuntia,* a cactus, are quick
to colonize exposed soil, and both are resistant to drought and to
the attacks of herbivorous animals. *Tridax procumbens* occurs almost
everywhere where man has disturbed the soil and seems especially
well adapted to places where building operations are in progress.
It is one of the first species to colonize bare earth and once it has
done so it provides an excellent environment for additional colonizing species, including the common African monocotyledon,
Commelina. Opuntia has been effectively controlled in Australia,
where it was also introduced, by an insect, and although there are
no serious attempts to control it in Africa other than by cutting it
down, it seems possible that eventually a method of control similar
to that used in Australia will be tried in Africa.

With the possible exception of man himself, insects are by far the
biggest overall threat to economic development in tropical Africa.
There is an enormous diversity of species and many of them are (or
may become) threats to agriculture, and, because of the diseases
they carry, to human health and the health of livestock. At the same
time many insects are essential to agriculture as they consume pest
species, pollinate flowers, and decompose dead vegetation. With a
few exceptions most of the ecological information on the insects of
Africa concerns species that have been shown to be pests or to be
useful. Knowledge of the numerous potential pests is virtually non-
existent, indeed a high proportion of the species in some of the
groups have not even been named.

Insects that are agricultural pests may be divided into several
categories. There are those that feed directly on the leaves, stems,
flowers, and fruits of plants by chewing the tissue. They cause
damage that is easily seen. Then there are those that bore into
stems and woody tissue destroying the inside of the plant to such an
extent that the yield of the crop is substantially reduced. A third
category consists of insects that live on the surface of the plant but
insert the proboscis into the tissues, usually into the xylem, and
suck out the nutrients contained in the water. These are all members
of the Hemiptera and some of them extract large quantities of water
from the plant as well as amino acids that are essential for the
formation of protein. The sucking insects in particular often transmit diseases from plant to plant: their mode of feeding facilitates

the transfer of viruses and other organisms in much the same way as a biting fly transmits diseases from one animal to another. The most destructive insects are nearly all members of the orders Orthoptera (grasshoppers and locusts), Lepidoptera (the larvae of butterflies and moths), Coleoptera (adults and larvae of beetles), Diptera (especially the larvae that bore into stems), and Hemiptera (immature and adult bugs that extract juices from plants by sucking).

A tremendous amount of research is directed at controlling and eradicating insect pests, and there are large organizations that are concerned primarily with the control of only a handful of species. Thus the Centre for Overseas Pest Research in London has for many years initiated fundamental and applied research on locusts and other grasshoppers, and has taken part in the planning and implementation of control measures. Insects like locusts are international pests and organizations that are concerned with their control must necessarily be free to operate in a diverse array of different countries that are affected by the pests. This has sometimes proved difficult, and especially in recent years when national borders have become more difficult to cross and when many nations regard each other with suspicion. Much research is oriented towards the control of pest populations by the use of insecticides, an operation that sometimes creates more problems than it solves because of the contamination of the environment that often arises, and towards biological control; but in recent years there has been a growing feeling that many insects cannot be fully controlled and that the best solution is to adjust the agriculture accordingly (Geier, 1966). So far as the use of insecticides is concerned it is becoming increasingly apparent that many insects can rapidly evolve resistant strains to the effects of the poison, and the research worker is left with nothing more than the satisfaction that he has generated an evolutionary change.

Grasshoppers are especially abundant in the grassy savanna areas of tropical Africa. There are relatively few species in the forest, where grass is rare, and none of the forest species is really common. Locusts are grasshoppers whose numbers will under certain conditions build up to plague proportions and which will undertake long-distance movements often resulting in serious damage and complete devastation of crops, and indeed of almost all other vegetation. There are three species of locust in tropical Africa, the migratory locust, *Locusta migratoria*, the red locust, *Nomadacris septemfasciata*, and the desert locust, *Schistocerca gregaria*. Many other grass-hoppers from time to time cause more or less extensive damage to crops, but none of them is as yet as important as the three locusts. Almost every year additional species of grasshopper are being added to those that are already regarded as pests, and it can be predicted that this trend will continue, especially as cereal crops are planted on a larger scale. Thus *Oedaleus senegalensis* is a widespread grass-hopper in the semi-arid tropics of Africa, and in recent years there have been increasing numbers of reports of local build-ups of populations and damage to grain crops (Batten, 1969). Jago (1968) lists 215 species of grasshopper from Ghana alone; many of these have the potential of becoming pests. The extent and rate at which they will do so depends mainly on the rate at which more land is brought under cultivation and on what crops are developed. Many of the common grasshoppers occur chiefly in arid areas and it is of course in such areas that cultivation is at best a hazardous business because of the unreliable rainfall, and it would seem that the build-up of grasshopper populations to pest proportions will be most severely felt in the savanna.

The last plague of the migratory locust in tropical Africa began in 1928 and ended in 1941 (Batten, 1967). During this period the locust spread over much of Africa extending south to South Africa and east to the East African coast. The plague originated in the flood plains of the middle Niger in Mali (Lean, 1931) and its history over the years has been traced in detail. In West Africa there was a seasonal component to the movement of the swarms resulting from the parallel movement of the inter-tropical convergence zone, the locusts tending to be displaced southward and downwind, behaviour that has been recorded in other swarming locusts, especially the desert locust (Sayer, 1962). The southward movement of the migratory locust (and of the desert locust) that is associated with a wind from the north brings the swarms in October–December into areas that have recently had rain. The vegetation is therefore rela-tively lush and the moist conditions encourage breeding and hence more locusts. It thus appears that movements associated with the

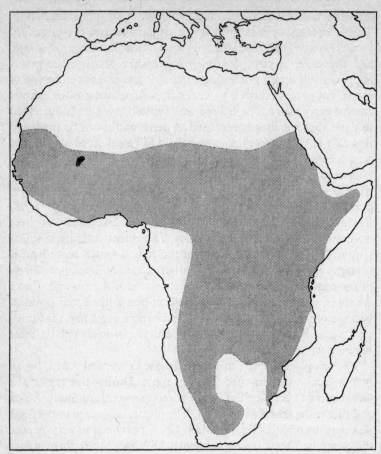

Fig. 5 Outbreak area (black) and invasion area (shaded) of the migratory locust in tropical Africa. (*Reproduced by permission of the Centre for Overseas Pest Research, London.*)

inter-tropical convergence front are not simply passive, but are adaptive in that the locusts are repeatedly displaced into more favourable areas. Fig. 5 shows the outbreak area of the migratory locust and the invasion area during recent plagues.

The outbreak areas of the red locust are in East Africa, and the most important is in the Rukwa Valley (Fig. 6). This locust breeds once a year and spends the long dry season in partial aestivation. In

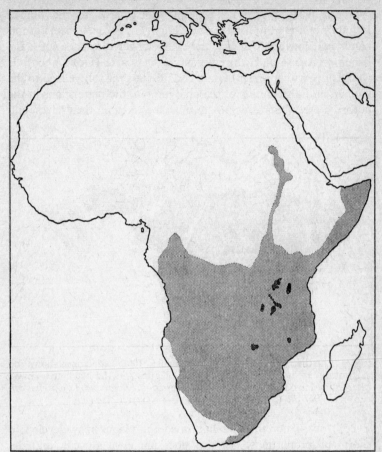

Fig. 6 Outbreak area (black) and invasion area (shaded) of the red locust during the last plague (1930–44). (*Reproduced by permission of the Centre for Overseas Pest Research, London.*)

most years the red locust is confined to the outbreak areas and thus attempts to prevent the development of plagues are concentrated on the insects within the outbreak areas (Yule, 1960; Woodrow, 1965; Symmons, *et al.*, 1963). Exactly what causes the red locust to build up in numbers and to move out of these areas is not fully understood, but they do so periodically and can invade almost the whole of the southern part of Africa, extending northwards to the Somali Republic and even to Madagascar. The nymphs, or 'hoppers', form bands and move downwind, travelling longer distances when the bands are dense and when vegetation is sparse (Dean, 1967). It would appear that under certain conditions, probably related to the amount and distribution of seasonal rainfall, the populations in the outbreak areas build-up and are unable to contain themselves, and

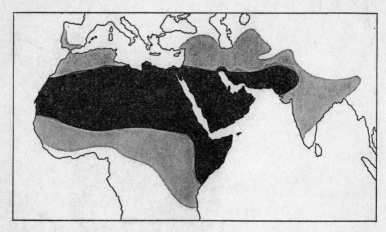

Fig. 7 The distribution of the desert locust. The shaded area shows the maximum extent of the locusts during plagues and the black area shows where they have been found during recessions. (*Reproduced by permission of the Centre for Overseas Pest Research, London.*)

so spill out. Once this has happened the plague may develop to enormous proportions, but this does not always occur, and the precise sequence of events after an initial outbreak is by no means predictable.

The desert locust is a much more serious potential pest than the other two species. It is not confined to outbreak areas of limited size, but may occur sporadically and in small numbers throughout a large part of the drier savanna and semi-desert north of the equator in Africa, and in Arabia and Pakistan (Fig. 7). The Red Sea coast has long been known as one of the most important places where plagues originate. With the build-up of populations in one or more of the many possible outbreak areas the locusts move in almost all directions, but usually downwind, and invade the whole of tropical Africa except the humid West Coast and the forested area of the Congo basin. The desert locust does not normally spread into the invasion area of the red locust, but a distinct subspecies occurs in South Africa which occasionally swarms, but which remains geographically separate from the northern subspecies (Botha, 1967). Damage to crops can be extensive and millions of people must have starved or have suffered extreme hardship as a result of the devastations of the desert locust. During times of recession it is sometimes difficult to ascertain the whereabouts of desert locusts in Africa and a few years ago when some live individuals were required for research purposes in Uganda they had to be imported from London where stocks are maintained in captivity. The ecology of the desert locust has been thoroughly investigated and there is a vast literature on almost all aspects of its biology. The information obtained serves as a model for research on other pest species and the essential features of what is known are outlined below.

Swarms of the desert locust are known to have occurred in North Africa and the Middle East since the beginnings of cultivation. It is particularly destructive to cereal crops and with the spread of cultivation of these crops into the savanna of tropical Africa the desert locust became an important threat to the lives of the cultivators. The possible invasion area extends over 26 million km^2 and over 110 degrees of longitude from West Africa to Assam and, at its widest, over 50 degrees of latitude from Turkey to southern Tanzania (Waloff, 1962). The chief characteristic of this enormous area, which is split into numerous nations and occupied by people of a wide array of political and religious beliefs, is that it is arid. Scattered through these arid regions are places where the locusts maintain themselves at rather low population densities, but under certain ecological conditions, notably of unseasonal or exceptional rainfall, the numbers build up, and after breeding there may be long distance displacements, some individual swarms moving up to 4000 km. Further breeding and movement may occur and the result is that the desert locust maintains itself in a permanent state of plague or potential plague.

The build-up and subsequent decline in numbers of the desert locust (and of some other species of locust) is associated with changes in the quality of the populations. When the locusts are at low density they exist in a phase which is known as *solitaria*, but as numbers increase there is a transition from this phase to what is known as *gregaria*. Individuals in the two phases differ markedly in behaviour, physiology, and morphology, and the stimulus to change from one phase to the other is a change in the density of the population, which in turn is usually associated with rainfall affecting the quantity and quality of the vegetation. It has long been realized that the key to understanding why locusts increase in numbers lies in understanding the nature of the phase variations. The differences between the two phases are listed in Table 17. Almost all the differences confer on *gregaria* a better potential to swarm and on *solitaria* the opposite effect. The most striking and obvious differences between the phases are in the coloration of the hoppers (Stower, 1959), but, when numbers are increasing, behavioural changes occur first, followed by colour change, and then by morphological changes (Roffey and Popov, 1968). There is evidence suggesting that *gregaria* individuals are far more resistant to drought and food deprivation than *solitaria* (Albrecht, 1962), and it has been proposed that the two phases represent a 'division of labour' within the population such that the *gregaria* individuals are best adapted to situations that favour high density, movement, and opportunism, while the *solitaria* individuals are adapted to a more stable environment and low population density (Kennedy, 1961). The important feature of the system is that one phase can be rapidly converted to the other and it is this that promotes the magnitude, irregularity, and unpredictability of the swarms.

The prevention of a build-up of locusts and subsequent plagues obviously depends on a detailed knowledge of what happens when *solitaria* is being converted to *gregaria*, and also of course where and when these changes are occurring. Much effort has been devoted to this and also to aerial spraying of swarms once they develop. It is not of course possible to estimate the effectiveness of control measures because it is never known what might have happened if no efforts at control had been made. The Centre for Overseas Pest Research is well aware of the difficulties in interpreting the results of the research that has been done and this is why it continues to expand its programme of training scientists in locust biology. At present there are indications of the development of another plague of desert locusts, and although more is known about this species than about any other insect pest, there remain numerous difficulties in making valid predictions as to exactly what is likely to happen in the future (Roffey, 1969). It looks as if spraying the swarms with insecticide has reduced numbers and prevented the build-up of plagues in some areas, notably in West Africa since 1961 (MacCuaig, 1963), and recent evidence that dieldrin can be transmitted to the offspring of locusts (Watts, 1969) perhaps provides the best hope that insecticides may play a significant role in the control of populations as the effects of the insecticide will be carried with the swarms from one place to another.

A wide variety of invertebrate and vertebrate predators and parasites are known to feed on the eggs, hoppers, and adults of the desert locust (Greathead, 1963, 1966; Stower and Greathead, 1969), but whether any of these can be used as a means of biological control is not known. Prospects seem poor, mainly because of the mobility of the swarms once they enter the *gregaria* phase. The same can be said of diseases, and although the discovery of an epidemic of a fungus disease has been reported (Balfour-Browne, 1960), it seems that prospects for its use as a means of controlling numbers are remote. But there are other possibilities that are currently being investigated. Gibberellic acid is necessary in the diet of the desert locust for fast maturation, and diets that are deficient in gibberellins, such as senescent vegetation, can produce diapause in the adults (Carlisle, et al., 1969; Ellis, et al., 1965). The possibility of producing a synthetic food that inhibits sexual maturation is being investigated, although exactly how such knowledge could be applied to a field situation is not entirely clear. In addition, maturation is stimulated in the desert locust after they have eaten the leaves or flowers of myrrh, *Commiphora* spp., plants of the family Burseraceae, which in the Somali peninsula become available just before the onset of the rain (Carlisle, et al., 1965). This being so it is possible that the absence of myrrh and other aromatic desert shrubs would lead to a failure of the locusts to synchronize their breeding with the rains, an event which stimulates the beginning of the transition from *solitaria* to *gregaria* and the subsequent build-up of the swarm.

It thus appears that the desert locust is likely to continue as a major threat to agriculture in the drier parts of Africa. Much is known about its biology and how it could be controlled. The major difficulty is the implementation of the knowledge. Both the red and the migratory locust are likely to be less of a threat in the future as their outbreak areas are rather small and it should be possible to monitor changes and to take appropriate action when and where there are indications of a rise in population size. The desert locust presents a more difficult problem as its outbreak area is scattered over millions of square kilometres of country.

The success of locusts as pests depends on their ability to expand out of restricted areas as their population density rises. It is possible that many other animals that have become pests of crops possess elements of this kind of behaviour, and two such animals, one a moth and the other a bird, are now being investigated by using the same approaches and techniques as have been used on locusts.

The army-worm is the larva of a noctuid moth, *Spodoptera exempta*. This and similar species occur throughout the savanna and cultivated areas of tropical Africa, and it is becoming apparent that the moths are migratory, the movements being more or less regular and therefore unlike those of locusts. At times the moth breeds in large numbers over a wide area and the resulting larvae are destructive to cereal crops and pasture grasses. An entire crop may fail as the result of the depredations of the larvae.

The weaver bird, *Quelea quelea*, is a small sparrow-like species that frequently reaches plague proportions in the drier parts of Africa (Fig. 8). It feeds chiefly on the seeds of grasses, including those of cereal crops, and is particularly abundant in the savanna areas of West and East Africa. According to Ward (1965) the economy of at least seventeen different countries can be affected by the destruction caused by this bird. In southern Mauritania an average density of 12 400 nests per hectare has been estimated and the birds utilize about 186 kg of grass per hectare for nest building and consume about 1845 kg of seeds per hectare during the short breeding season (Morel, 1968). They nest in dense colonies and after breeding roam the countryside in great flocks, settling wherever the seeds of grasses and cereal are ripening. Efforts to control their numbers have included the use of flame throwers to destroy the

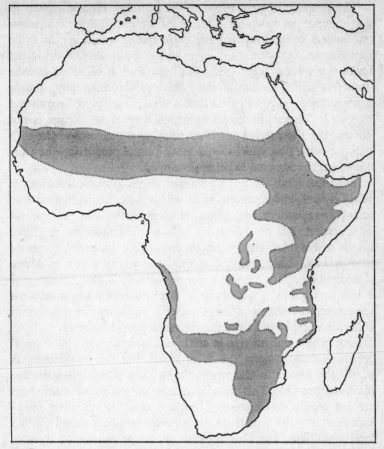

Fig. 8. Area of Africa liable to invasion by *Quelea* birds. (*Reproduced by permission of the Centre for Overseas Pest Research, London.*)

nests. It has been estimated that 80 million birds were destroyed during programmes of control in Senegal in 1959 and 60 million around Lake Chad in Northern Nigeria, and yet despite these efforts there is no evidence of a substantial decrease in numbers (Ward, 1965). Indeed as more and more savanna is cultivated with cereals the ecological conditions of the bird are improving and it can be predicted that it will continue to increase and cause severe damage to crops.

The build-up of large roosts of the fruit bat, *Eidolon helvum*, in and around the towns of tropical Africa and the periodic mass movements of the bats that use these roosts, would appear to be partly associated with the changes in the availability of cultivated fruits upon which they feed. The bats feed at night on a wide variety of fruits, both wild and cultivated (Mutere, 1967), but in general they seem to take fruit that is already too ripe to be gathered by people. Hence the extent to which they cause damage is not known, but the species possesses many of the characteristics of a highly mobile pest which could reach plague proportions in areas where fruit production is being developed.

The pests of all the more important crops in tropical Africa are relatively well-known and in areas where plantation agriculture for cash crops occurs there are fairly efficient methods of pest control in operation. But of course the bulk of the cultivation in Africa occurs where there are few resources available for possible control measures to be implemented. Almost every crop grown in Africa is affected by a broad spectrum of pests, most of them insects, and a wide variety of diseases, many of them transmitted by insects. In the account that follows I have selected three crops, rice, cocoa, and coffee, in order to illustrate the problems caused by pests.

Swamp and upland rice is cultivated in many areas of tropical Africa, especially along the West Coast, but the productivity is nearly the lowest in the world, being only about one-sixth the maximum possible. This is partly because the methods of cultivation are not highly developed and because there is still little information as to which of the many varieties are best suited for the local conditions, but also because of the prevalence of diseases caused by funguses, viruses, and bacteria, and the damage caused by insects, weaver birds, and rodents. The diseases and pests of rice and the methods by which they may be controlled are summarized in a manual produced by the (British) Ministry of Overseas Development (1970), from which the account that follows is taken.

Of the fungal diseases, blast caused by *Pyricularia oryzae* is the most important. It affects the leaves and the stems and is most serious when the neck region of the flowering stem is attacked; the tissues of the stem rot and the panicle falls over. Many varieties of *P. oryzae* exist which differ in physiology and each seems to be adapted to a particular strain of rice. Some varieties of rice are more resistant to blast than others, and in areas where the disease is prevalent such strains are being encouraged. In the 1930s when rice was being developed as a crop in Sierra Leone, blast was not considered an important disease, but with the expansion of rice cultivation it became evident that the disease was spreading. Other fungal diseases of rice cause the rot or blight of the leaves and stems, and a general weakening of the plants as well as the failure to produce seeds.

Bacterial and virus diseases of rice occur in tropical Africa, but little is known of their distribution or of their effect on the crop. This is partly because there are so few people working in the field who are competent to identify the diseases, let alone initiate programmes of control. The virus diseases are mainly transmitted by leaf-hoppers, Hemiptera, that suck the juices from the leaves and stems of the growing plants. Nematodes occur in almost all plants and most species alternate a soil phase with a phase that lives on the plant. In Africa several species have been identified as causing damage to rice plants, among them *Aphelenchoides besseyi*, an ectoparasite that feeds on the young and unfurled leaves causing them to wither and droop. Nematodes pierce the cell walls of the plant tissue and the damage caused in this way provides a site for infection with funguses and bacteria. The effect of nematodes is thus twofold. Other species of nematode attack the roots of rice and their general effect is to inhibit the growth of the plant. Amphibious snails attack the germinating seeds and very young plants and sometimes destroy them in great numbers. Shrimps and crabs cause similar damage, and in West Africa the crab *Sesarma huzardi* attacks the newly transplanted seedlings in tidal mangrove swamps cutting them off at ground level (Jordan, 1957).

But the principal threat to rice production in Africa and elsewhere in the world is the damage caused by insects. Insect pests of rice can be divided into four types: stem-borers, plant suckers, leaf feeders, and stem and root feeders. The most important stem-borers are the larvae of moths belonging to the families Noctuidae and Pyralidae. The adult moths lay their eggs on the stems and upon hatching the larvae bore inside and feed on the soft tissues. The growth of the plant is retarded and the stems topple over because of the destruction of the supporting tissue and the interruption of the nutrient flow. There may be many larvae on one plant, but most plants contain only a few larvae. More than one species of borer may infect a plant at a time. Stalk-eyed flies, Diopsidae, are similar pests. The larvae bore into the stems and consume the inner tissues of the plant. At times the adult flies can be extremely abundant, and I have seen great swarms of one species in rice fields in Sierra Leone. Plant suckers are all members of the Hemiptera. They extract water and nutrients from the plant and when they are common they inhibit growth and are also responsible for transmitting viruses. The leaf feeders are chiefly the larvae of moths, and the adults and nymphs of grasshoppers, including the three species of locust already discussed. They feed directly on the leaves, especially at or near the growing points of the plant, and thus reduce the photosynthetic area of the plant as well as changing the normal pattern of growth. The stem and root feeders are chiefly the larvae of Diptera and Coleoptera, but include mole crickets, *Gryllotalpa*, which are Orthoptera. The most important root and stem feeder is *Pachydiplosis oryzae*, the rice gall midge, a member of the dipterous family Cecidomyiidae. At times almost the entire crop can be lost through the attacks of this insect.

Rice suffers an enormous amount of damage from weaver birds which not only eat the seeds but also take the leaves for nest building. In the drier areas *Quelea quelea* may devastate the crop, while similar but less extensive damage is caused by the related *Ploceus cucullatus* in the wetter areas of West and Central Africa. Some migrant birds from Europe and Asia feed on rice seedlings and newly planted seed. Among these is the ruff, *Philomachus pugnax*, which in Europe feeds on invertebrates, and is protected by conservationists because of its beauty and unusual breeding behaviour, but while wintering in Africa can cause extensive damage by removing planted rice seeds.

Among the extraordinary diversity of species of rodents that occur in West Africa (Rosevear, 1969) there are within restricted areas a few species that are particularly common while most are rather rare. Many rodents feed on the leaves and seeds of wild grasses and the creation of rice fields has provided an excellent environment for high population densities.

Much rice is lost during storage. The crop is one that is frequently stored in rural African villages, and there are usually heavy losses during the period of storage (in most areas the dry season) through moulds, beetle larvae, and rodents.

These are some of the more important natural hazards to the cultivation of rice. Other pests and diseases are known, and it seems certain that as more rice is grown these will have increasing effects on the production of the crop.

Virtually all the rice grown in Africa is for local consumption, but cocoa is an important cash crop and most of what is produced is exported. The main producing countries are Ghana, Nigeria, Cameroon, and the Ivory Coast. The trees have to grow for three or four years before producing the first crop and they may live for more than sixty years. They are grown either in plantations or by local cultivators. Cocoa is a forest crop and the conditions under which it is grown are similar to those that occur in primary rain forest. Under such circumstances it is not astonishing that cocoa is attacked by numerous pests, most of which are insects, and is affected by several insect-borne diseases. The literature on the insect associations that occur on cocoa farms is reviewed by Leston (1970) who also gives a commendably lively summary of the problems encountered by illiterate people faced with modern methods of dealing with insect pests. The most important pests of cocoa are bugs of the family Miridae, frequently called cocoa-capsids. Several species occur in West and Central Africa where cocoa is grown and the main damage is caused by the bugs sucking the new tissue near the growing points of the trees, but they also transmit fungus diseases (Entwistle, 1964). In Ghana the capsids and the fungus they introduce probably reduce the potential crop by 20 per cent. *Distantiella*, the most numerous of the West African cocoa-capsids, was at first controlled quite effectively by spraying the trees with insecticides, but it developed resistant strains (Dunn, 1963), and according to Leston (1970) the post-independence breakdown of extension services in Ghana thwarted the continuation of attempts to control the pest.

In West Africa about twenty species of mealy-bugs (Hemiptera) feed on cocoa and many of them transmit swollen shoot virus which is extremely destructive to cocoa. Leston (1970) reports that between

1947 and 1957 about 70 million trees were cut down in Ghana in attempts to control the virus and it is possible that the better cocoa crops in the early 1960s were the result of this campaign. Mealy-bugs are attended by ants and some species cannot survive without the presence of ants. Other species of ants are predators of the mealy-bugs and of capsids, and their presence on the cocoa farms may be more effective in controlling bug populations than spraying with insecticide. During the spraying the ants are also killed and this in some circumstances could lead to a rise in the mealy-bug and capsid population sizes. Leston (1970) suggests that it would be possible to increase cocoa production tenfold by creating a competent extension service and by growing the cocoa under plantation conditions with adequate equipment and skilled man-power, but raises the question as to whether this is wise when the world market for the product is so uncertain. Leston concludes that 'we are left, therefore, with no choice but to support the present small farms and to continue recommending this or that formulation to farm labourers who cannot read what's on the tin'.

Coffee occupies a similar position in the economy of East Africa as cocoa in West Africa. But it will grow under a wider range of ecological conditions and considerable quantities are produced throughout Africa. In Kenya and elsewhere there are large coffee plantations producing good quality berries. These plantations are under skilled management and in general the efficiency of produc-tion is high. But in many areas, notably in Uganda, the bulk of the coffee is produced by small farmers, who do not have the capital and knowledge to initiate pest control programmes and it is under these conditions that the effects of diseases and pests are likely to be economically devastating.

Many different species of insect have been recorded from coffee and the importance of each varies with the area in which the coffee is being grown and with the variety of coffee grown (Schmutterer, 1969). Most of the important pests are the larvae of moths. These insects have moved on to coffee from related wild species and as more and more coffee is grown the impact of these pests is increas-ing. One of these moths is the coffee leaf miner, *Leucoptera meyricki*, a member of the family Lyonetiidae. It was at one time considered an insignificant pest, but has in recent years reached high densities and caused severe damage to coffee in Kenya. The change in the moth's status as a pest is associated with two changes in the growing of coffee. First, the practice of mulching which favours the growth of the coffee bush provides a better environment for the pupation of the larvae, and secondly, the increased frequency of spraying with copper fungicides produces a better leaf and a more favourable environment for the larvae of the moth which bore into leaf tissue (Crowe, 1964). Thus it seems that two operations designed to improve the coffee bushes have resulted in an increase of a pest species. It is now suggested that if spraying is restricted to a certain stage in the life cycle of the moth it can be effective, but the situation illustrates remarkably well what is probably of common occurrence: efforts designed to reduce the effect of one pest or disease may result in the increase of another. There is a further complication in that spraying tends to kill the parasites of the leaf miner and here again restriction of the spraying operations to certain phases of the life cycle is recommended (Bess, 1964; Wheatley and Crowe, 1964).

The green looper, *Epigynopteryx stictigramma*, is the larva of a moth of the family Geometridae. The larvae feed on the leaves of coffee and until quite recently were not regarded as serious pests. Recent outbreaks have been associated with the application of an insecticide to reduce the numbers of the leaf miner. The insecticide seems to kill the natural parasites of the green looper and numbers then rise as the larger looper larvae appear to be unaffected by the insecticide (Crowe and Leeuwangh, 1965; Leeuwangh, 1965). Other insecticides, including DDT, have been suggested as a possible means of controlling the green looper, but it is known that the application of DDT can lead to outbreaks of other pests, including mealy-bugs and lacebugs, probably because of the selective removal of their natural enemies. Besides eating the leaves, berries, and flowers of coffee, the green looper produces wounds in the plant tissue that give access for a fungus that causes leaf blight.

The coffee berry borer, *Hypothenemus hampei*, is a beetle of the family Scolytidae and it has been found that in Uganda this pest can bore into as many as 90 per cent of the berries (Ingram, 1968), although not all the bored berries are unfit for use. It is believed that spraying can reduce the numbers of the pest, but in view of the experience with the leaf miner and the green looper, large-scale spraying must be watched carefully because of possible increases in other pests. Another serious pest in East Africa is the bug, *Antestiopsis lineaticollis*, a member of the Pentatomidae, and a search is being made to find parasites that might be used in its biological control (Greathead, 1969), although as discussed earlier in this chapter, this is at best a hazardous business.

This account of coffee and its pests and diseases could be extended. Many other insects attack coffee and many difficulties have been encountered in trying to decide exactly how the numerous problems should be overcome. Coffee, like all tropical African cash crops, is attacked by numerous insects, and the diversity of species involved tends to frustrate rather than encourage control by either chemical or biological means.

The termites are among the more distinctive and conspicuous insects that are encountered in tropical Africa. They occur everywhere and play an important role in the functioning of natural and man-made ecosystems. Termites belong to the insect order Isoptera. They live in organized societies divided into different castes each of which has a distinct ecological (and social) role. Termites feed essentially on dead vegetation, especially wood and grass, the colonies formed are dispersed and food is obtained away from the colony but is brought back to be eaten, digested, and defecated. This means that nutrients are collected from a wide area but are eventually deposited within the limited area of the colony. Much of the food taken consists of cellulose; symbiotic Protozoa, bacteria, and funguses are associated with the breakdown of the cellulose.

Termites are so numerous in tropical Africa that they must constitute one of the most important decomposers of dead vegetation. They become pests when they attack timber used in building or wood that is being prepared for use. Wood is often transported over long distances for local use and this results in species of termites being introduced into many areas where previously they had been absent. They have for instance been repeatedly introduced into northern Europe but the climate prevents their survival. Termites are particularly damaging to plantations of *Eucalyptus* trees (Harris, 1961, 1966). *Eucalyptus* trees of a variety of species have been introduced into Africa from Australia and reports of damage to the roots and bark of these trees have come from Nigeria, Cameroon,

and The Gambia. Indeed in Sierra Leone it is often possible to
identify a *Eucalyptus* tree by the extensive damage caused by
termites to the bark.

The vegetation pattern of some areas of savanna is partly determined by the dispersion of termite colonies. The mounds formed
by the colonies tend to concentrate humus and nitrogen and this in
turn affects the species and abundance of plants, giving rise to the
distinctive clumps of vegetation that occur in many savanna areas
(Glover *et al.*, 1964).

Most attempts to control termites involve the application of
insecticides. But widespread control could lead to changes in the
energy balance of an ecosystem, particularly by slowing down the
rate of decomposition and allowing an accumulation of dead
vegetation. This could have effects on agriculture, although, it
must be admitted, the role of termites in the nutrient and energy
cycles of the soil has not as yet been properly investigated.

From what has been said in this chapter it should be evident that
human ecology is intimately bound up with the ecology of insects.
Everywhere insects dominate the scene and their effects on man's
attempts to cultivate are complex and in general poorly understood.
Almost all the research on insects has been directed at specific
known pests or at specific crops. As has been shown in the case of
coffee, the control of one pest can lead to an increase in the destruc-
tiveness of another. Insects and weeds have a short generation time
and this together with their high population densities provides much
scope for evolutionary change. Many examples of the evolution of
resistance to control measures, especially to the effects of insecticides,
have been documented, and there seems little doubt that in the
future more and more adaptive responses will be discovered as man
continues to struggle with methods of control. Complete control of
pests is probably impossible, and even in situations where a high
degree of control is possible, there are economic dangers in producing more of a cash crop than the uncertain world market can
accommodate.

Mention has been made of possibilities of controlling insect pests
by genetic means. Research is now proceeding in this direction, in
attempts to control not only agricultural pests but also species that
transmit diseases to man and his domestic animals. It also seems

that it will be possible to control some insect pests by regulating physiological processes, such as growth, development, and maturation, by the use of hormones (Ellis, 1968). Insects possess several hormones that control their development from egg to adult and alteration of the effect of a hormone at a critical stage in the life cycle could conceivably leave the insect as a permanent juvenile.

As more and more of the long-established ecosystems of tropical areas are destroyed and the land cultivated, insects will become adapted to the new circumstances. The most obvious adaptation is the transfer from one group of wild food plants to a group of cultivated plants and their weeds. Many examples of this are already known. Thus the larvae of the citrus swallowtail butterfly, *Papilio demodocus*, have become almost completely adapted to eating the leaves of introduced citrus plants. They formerly fed on wild species of Rutaceae and there is evidence that not only have they moved to citrus but are in the process of exploiting other food plants, including introduced species of Compositae. The closely related and possibly conspecific *Papilio demoleus* of Australia feeds on a member of the Leguminosae and there is evidence that it is just beginning to move to citrus (Wilson, 1965). These butterflies and other insects like them should provide interesting information on the capacity of insects to adapt to the rapidly changing environment that has occurred with the invention and spread of agriculture, and with the measures taken to protect crops from pests and diseases.

Lastly, it is odd that although some African animals have been introduced into other parts of the world and have become serious pests, these animals have not become pests in Africa itself, despite the ecological changes brought about by agriculture. The best known example is the giant snail, *Achatina fulica*, still confined to the East African coast, and yet a major pest of cultivation in many parts of tropical Asia and the Pacific region where it has been introduced by man (Mead, 1961). There is an ecological problem here that would be worth elucidating.

CHAPTER 7

Wild and Domestic Animals

The grasslands of the African savanna have until recent times supported enormous concentrations of large herbivorous mammals and their associated predators. The spectacular disappearance of these mammals from much of Africa in the past hundred years or so has been caused by the rapid expansion of human populations and by the careless slaughter carried out by Europeans earlier in the present century. Large concentrations of mammals can nowadays be seen only in areas set aside as national parks and in a few remote places that thus far have remained unpopulated. There is evidence that during the Pleistocene man hunted these mammals for food, and it is also likely that the presence of large mammals in abundance inhibited the early development of agriculture in Africa.

Evidence from hand axes suggests that about 50 000 years ago man was widely distributed in Africa and it was about this time that many genera of large mammals suddenly became extinct. It has often been proposed that climatic change (always invoked when no other explanation can be found) was responsible for this remarkable and sudden extinction of species and genera of African mammals, but Martin (1966, 1967) has persuasively argued that early man was responsible. A similarly rapid extinction occurred considerably later in North America with the arrival of the incipient Indians from Asia, and in Madagascar about 1000 years ago with the arrival of people from Melanesia. After the extinction of many kinds of mammals in Africa about 50 000 years ago, the remaining species may have increased in abundance and remained common until both the Europeans and the greatly expanded negroid populations began to destroy them systematically with firearms. But in addition to the direct effects of man, the wild mammals have increasingly suffered through competition with cattle and other domesticated animals.

Several thousand years ago pastoralism was widespread in what is now the Sahara Desert, and in all probability the pastoralists were forced south into the northern savanna as the desert began to dry up. The Nilotic people of the upper Nile had (and still have) large numbers of cattle, and it is believed that with the drying up of the area they moved south into Uganda and Kenya and became the Acholi, Langi, and Luo, some of whom still keep cattle while others have become cultivators. The Nilo-Hamites, represented today by numerous tribes, including the Karamojong of Uganda and the Turkana of Kenya, have probably been pastoralists for a long time, and many other Nilo-Hamitic groups of East Africa are today partly pastoralists and partly cultivators, while some have become entirely adapted to the growing of crops. Among all these people cattle are held in almost religious esteem and as a result many pastoralists run short of food in years of drought because they have failed to plant subsistence crops. When this happens they are forced to trade their cattle for food produced by nearby cultivators.

Pastoralists are traditionally nomadic and as their numbers and the numbers of their cattle increase they are having an ever-increasing effect on the grassland environment and upon the wild mammals that live in this environment. One of the major problems for present-day conservationists is the spread of pastoralists and their cattle into areas that have been set aside for the conservation of the large mammals. As will be shown later in this chapter this has generated much discussion and disagreement. One of the problems encountered by the conservationists is that pastoralists like the Masai have little concept of land tenure, at least not as it is understood by the conservationists. All land is considered as open grazing and its limits are defined only in terms of what can be reached by a nomadic group. But despite this there is a marked understanding within a large group that specific areas are more or less reserved for certain segments of the group. This understanding seems to work well as far as the Masai are concerned but it creates problems for others interested in alternative uses for the land. Apart from the conservationists the main threat to the Masai is the spread of the cultivators, although there are of course ecological differences between the two ways of life which result in a division of the land, based mainly on the amount and seasonal distribution of the rainfall: the requirements of cattle are not identical to those of cassava.

The term savanna is used to include a wide variety of habitats, but all share some common features, including the presence of grasses, the occurrence of one or two long dry seasons, and the susceptibility of the grass to extensive burning. Savanna areas may be devoid of trees, there may be a more or less continuous tree cover (although the trees are always well spaced), or there may be clumps of shrubby vegetation originating from mounds created by termites of the genus *Macrotermes*. The production of new grass usually begins just before the onset of the seasonal rains, especially if there has been a fire, and reaches its peak towards the end of the rains and early in the dry season. At the height of the dry season the grass dies and the landscape is brown and dead-looking. The alternation of wet and dry seasons dominates the life of the savanna pastoralist and his animals, and indeed the lives of all other organisms, including the numerous invertebrates that are vectors of disease. When plant production is at its peak there is an abundance of food, but in the dry season food may become scarce, and in addition the availability of water becomes a critical factor.

There have been numerous studies of savanna ecosystems in Africa, but there is so much variation in the structure of the savanna from place to place that generalizing is difficult. Vesey-Fitzgerald (1963) in an analysis of the grasslands of the Rukwa Valley in south-west Tanzania and northern Zambia, distinguishes between grass-land that has not been extensively modified by man and secondary grassland which originated and is maintained by circumstances induced by man, especially by annual burning. In secondary grass-lands regeneration is often maintained in a subclimax state by fire or some other factor induced by man. There are some people who feel that virtually all the savanna of Africa is secondary.

In many areas there are extensive patches of grassland composed of a single dominant species, but the particular species present will depend on the kind of soil, the biological effectiveness of the rainfall, and the amount of grazing pressure from wild and domesticated animals, as well as the regularity and intensity of seasonal fires. The woody vegetation (if present) often consists of species that are more or less fire-resistant, and many of the trees and shrubs are also resistant to grazing by mammals, mainly because they possess thorns or toxic compounds that make them unpalatable.

Grassland fires can start from lightning during dry thunder-storms, but this is probably rather unusual, and most fires are started by man. It is not known for how long the savanna of Africa has been subjected to burning in the dry season, but it seems that fires date from before the expansion of the negroid populations, and the ability to use fire was known to the earlier bushmen of southern Africa (Clark, 1951). Many insects have evolved adaptive responses to seasonal fires and this alone suggests that the phenomenon is quite ancient. In the last few centuries the burning of the grassland has become universal and almost every area is burnt over at least once a year during the dry season. Attempts to prohibit burning in the national parks where large mammals are protected have met with only limited success: much of the grassland in Queen Elizabeth National Park is burnt over about once a year and it appears that no one can do anything to stop this. It seems as if setting fire to dead vegetation is part of the African way of life for it is not only in the savanna but also in cultivated areas that vegetation is set alight as soon as it is dry. There has been much discussion of the good and bad effects of grassland burning, and there is no consensus, except that under certain circumstances it is good and under others it is bad. It seems to me likely that it depends on one's point of view, and in any case from the ecological point of view it is irrelevant whether it is good or bad; what is important is that it happens.

Most of the really large savanna fires are deliberately started by pastoralists at the end of the dry season. The fire destroys dead vegetation and probably arthropod vectors of disease (and countless other invertebrates), and encourages the grass to sprout new leaves, which can then be utilized by the hungry cattle. On the whole fire is less destructive than cultivation as the plants that grow up after the fire are in general the same species that were there before, whereas after cultivation complex successional patterns are gener-ated, often involving colonization by what might be regarded as weed species. As far as the pastoralists are concerned burning the vegetation is a most useful practice. Pastoralists are more difficult to administer and control than cultivators, and their individuality would suggest that no matter what governments and experts pro-pound about the long-term effects of fire on the landscape, they will happily continue setting alight any patch of dead grass they happen to encounter. Some people maintain that over a large area of Africa the hydrological cycle has been seriously affected by fire, chiefly by increasing the rate of surface evaporation and hence lowering the water table. Sparse vegetation has been converted into desert and relatively lush savanna into dry bush, while there is much evidence of the spread of savanna-like conditions into areas that were until recently humid rain forest. The Sahara Desert is said to be advancing at a rate of several kilometres a year along a 3200 km front (Allan, 1965) and in recent years attention has repeatedly been drawn to the spread of desert and semi-desert conditions throughout the northern part of East Africa. But apart from fire the increasing grazing pressure exerted by cattle will in itself reduce the amount of vegetation and hasten the drying up process. Wild mammals confined to national parks are thought to encourage the retreat of forest and the spread of grassland, and hence the spread of fires, but there is no agreement as to exactly what role the larger mammals play in this matter.

The effects of savanna fires are felt even along the humid West African coast. At times great palls of smoke drift southwards and this together with dust makes the atmosphere very unpleasant. The role of fire as an atmospheric pollutant has scarcely been considered, but it would seem likely that the health of both people and animals is affected by the amount of smoke in the air, which apparently increases every year. And yet there seems nothing that can be done to stop the fires, even if anyone seriously wanted to stop them on a large scale. As mentioned earlier pastoralists are not easy people to govern, and most administrators prefer to leave them alone; in any case they inhabit areas that must be written off in terms of development, except where they infringe on the programmes of conservation of mammals for aesthetic and scientific purposes.

It is likely that the African grasslands have been heavily grazed for thousands of years, but since their introduction cattle have steadily replaced the wild mammals as consumers of grass. Evidently the different species of grass-feeding mammals select both different species of grass and the different component parts of grass. Thus in the Serengeti National Park in Tanzania several species of grazing mammals, including the zebra, wildebeest, and topi, migrate through the area at different times and each species exploits different parts of the available grass (Gwynne and Bell, 1968). There is a marked difference in the frequency of leaves, sheaths, and stems in the diet of the three species, as shown in Table 18. In the case of the wildebeest and the zebra there are also differences between the wet and the dry seasons in the parts of the grass taken. The zebra in particular is able to utilize the stems of grasses and since it is the first to migrate through the area it opens up the herb layer and increases the frequency of available leaves which are utilized by the wildebeest, the next migrant to pass through the area. The topi is a partial migrant and its feeding habits are intermediate between those of the zebra and the wildebeest. Thomson's gazelle, which is also present in the area, feeds to a large extent on dicotyledons, including their fruits. It is the last to migrate through the area and because of this it can exploit more of the dicotyledon food which has been exposed by the grazing and trampling of the other species.

It has frequently been argued that wild grazers are less likely to destroy the grassland than cattle because each species is something of a specialist in its food requirements. There are a priori reasons for supposing that this argument is valid. First, the wild mammals have evolved in the savanna ecosystem and there has been much time for them to adapt to the special conditions of the savanna, the evolution of which as an ecosystem has been partly determined by selective pressures exerted by the grazers. Secondly, the species of wild mammals differ in their structure and physiology and it is thus likely that each is able to exploit efficiently a relatively narrow range of the available food. The differences between the species are themselves the result of interspecific competition for food. And thirdly, their numbers have until recently been regulated in a natural way by the pressures exerted by predators and by fluctuations in the availability of food. It would therefore seem that until man began to 'manage' the wild mammals their numbers were regulated in a density-dependent way like those of other wild populations. They are better adapted to the savanna than man's cattle, and it has been suggested that some of the existing cattle should be replaced by wild mammals, an idea that has considerable scientific merit, but which is unlikely to be acceptable to the pastoralists.

The main areas of Africa that support large numbers of cattle are arid and unsuitable for intensive cultivation. The wet season is short, but when there is rain there is plenty of fresh grass, although its quality is lower than that of European pastures, being rather less well supplied with nutrients. But most of the year the cattle are forced to graze on what has been termed 'standing hay' (Williamson and Payne, 1965), which in effect is dead grass that is still standing. Needless to say the quality of this food is low, and in particular it contains little protein because of the lack of green leaves and the abundance of fibrous material. Not only is food rather scarce but it is also of low digestibility, and this partly accounts for the poor quality of most of the savanna cattle, especially towards the end of the long dry season when the quality and quantity of the food available may be very low indeed. Biochemical tests have shown that Gambian cattle suffer from protein deficiency (Walshe and Gilles, 1962) and this is probably so elsewhere in Africa.

Cattle belong to the family Bovidae, and most domesticated kinds used in the world today belong either to the species *Bos taurus*, the common European type, or to *Bos indicus*, commonly known as the zebu, and the most frequent type in the tropics. There are numerous breeds of both of these so-called species, including hybrids between them. In Europe, North America, and elsewhere cattle have been selectively bred to produce animals that provide high yields of meat and milk, selection usually being for one or other of these qualities and not for both. In Africa cattle are also a source of food, but in many areas this is secondary to the function they play in social custom, religion, and as evidence of wealth and status. Partly because of this, breeding has been much more haphazard, the main consideration being the selection of kinds that are resistant to the environment, especially to disease and drought. Many African cattle thus appear to be of low quality compared with those of temperate regions, but they are well-adapted to the environment and serve their dual function extremely well.

Williamson and Payne (1965) discuss the origin of the different kinds of cattle that now occur in Africa, basing their account on an earlier publication by Payne. It appears that the original kinds were two distinct breeds of *Bos taurus* called the Hamitic longhorn and the shorthorn, and that these repeatedly mixed with *Bos indicus*, the zebu, to produce the Sanga cattle, which in various forms are the dominant breed throughout Africa today. Nearly pure strains of the two founder species are still to be found in some areas. Thus a breed similar to the Hamitic longhorn known as N'Dama occurs along the coast of the Gulf of Guinea where it can survive in forest areas presumably because it is relatively resistant to trypanosomiasis. Indeed the history of breeding cattle in Africa and the subsequent spread of different breeds can be understood largely in the context of which kinds are more resistant to trypanosomiasis and to other diseases. Zebu cattle in particular are more resistant to rinderpest than Sanga cattle and they do well in arid areas. There is some evidence that today the various breeds of zebu are still spreading and are replacing the Sanga cattle. This spread is to be expected as many savanna areas are becoming depleted of their vegetation through the action of cattle and the zebu can apparently survive in much harsher conditions than some of the other kinds.

Probably there are now over 100 million cattle in tropical Africa and their numbers, like those of the people, are increasing extremely rapidly. They have almost replaced the indigenous mammals. Conservationists around the world, alarmed at the reduction in numbers of the African wild mammals, have advocated that attempts should be made to farm them and that, at least in some areas, the wild mammals should be allowed to re-populate the areas now grazed by cattle. These wild mammals, it is argued, could be cropped and could be a better source of animal protein than the scraggy cattle that seem to occur everywhere. In addition they can be used as a tourist attraction, and can bring in money to governments by the development of the tourist industry. There is no doubt that large herds of wild mammals, such as can now be seen in the national parks of East and South Africa, are an important source of revenue from tourists, but there are several problems associated with farming wild mammals that do not appear to have been resolved, and in some cases not even discussed.

There are two conflicting interests: those of the cattle owners who live in the area and who in general are not concerned with world events, and those of the conservationists who do not usually live in the area but who are acquainted with the ecological problems created by over-grazing, and with the scientific and aesthetic value of large mammals. As already mentioned, most of the people that own cattle in Africa not only use them as a source of food, but also value them for social and religious reasons. A pastoralist's herd is to him a symbol of status which can be used in his own community for enhancing his prestige in much the same way as more affluent people acquire and operate an expensive car which they cannot really afford. It would be extremely difficult and most unreasonable to try to persuade cattle owners that they do not need so many cattle, and that they should instead look after a few antelope, just as it would be to persuade a business man that he does not need such a big car and that a smaller and more economical make would be better. Thus if the conservationists are going to succeed in replacing cattle with antelope they will have to face this problem, unless of course pastoralism is compulsorily replaced by ranch farming, an event which seems unlikely in the foreseeable future.

Cattle have been selectively bred by man for thousands of years and there is much knowledge as to how breeds of cattle can be improved to meet the peculiar conditions of an environment for which they are intended. Selective breeding has reached a high degree of sophistication in Europe and elsewhere, while in Africa it has probably proceeded on a trial and error basis with the result that the cattle that now live in Africa are the product of an evolutionary process in which the best types have been fitted to the environment. Nothing is known about the genetics of wild antelope or of other herbivorous mammals, and, moreover, there does not appear to be any attempt to find out if they can be selectively bred so as to increase their yields of meat and, especially, of milk. They have clearly evolved a considerable amount of natural immunity to disease, but this in itself will not make them desirable to the pastoralists. And then it could be disputed whether the domestication of wild mammals will really help in solving the problems of protein malnutrition. The shortage of protein is felt most in areas where cultivators grow cassava and other root crops, and not so much in the savanna where cattle are available. Thus if wild mammals are to be used to improve the nutrition of the people there must also be an improvement in the packaging and transportation of meat and milk to areas where the need is greatest.

Except in the national parks the wild mammals of Africa are decreasing rapidly. They are hunted and their environment is being destroyed by man and his cattle. In the national parks they are abundant and in some areas of East Africa it has been felt necessary to crop them to prevent over-grazing and subsequent erosion of the soil. The increase in abundance in the parks is probably the result of their present inability to undertake long distance movements as the food becomes locally depleted. Much time and money has been spent on research as to how the wild mammal populations can be maintained in enclosed or protected areas without serious destruction of the habitat, but although many points of view have emerged there is regrettably no general agreement as to how this should be done. Thus in Tsavo National Park in Kenya some research workers have advocated fairly intensive cropping of the elephant population, while others have argued that the apparent damage caused by the elephants is largely because of a succession of unusually dry years and is therefore of a temporary nature.

African cattle probably suffer from more diseases than those in other parts of the world. There is an enormous literature on the diseases of cattle, especially on trypanosomiasis and its insect vector, various species of tsetse flies, *Glossina*. Trypanosomiasis has recently been discussed in a book of 950 pages (Mulligan, 1971) which in itself indicates the amount of work that has been put into research on this disease. It has been found virtually impossible for cattle to survive in some parts of Africa because of the prevalence of trypanosomiasis. Indeed the destruction of the forest region of Africa might have taken place even more quickly had it not been for this disease, which affects man as well as cattle. The disease is caused by a variety of species, or strains, of *Trypanosoma*, and is transmitted by the tsetse fly when sucking blood from the host animal. Nearly all the species of wild mammals of Africa, as well as some other vertebrates, are infected (Ashcroft, 1959), and the disease has thus been transferred to cattle by flies that bite other animals and then cattle. Many of the wild mammals have acquired a natural immunity or partial immunity to the disease and so have some breeds of cattle. The disease may be treated with drugs and some progress is now being made with an effective vaccine, but despite intensive research there are still immense difficulties involved in ridding Africa of trypanosomiasis (Lumsden, 1967). Another approach has been to try and control the tsetse fly populations and various projects in different parts of Africa have been aimed at

9 The Pyrethrum Marketing Board's processing and refining complex at Nakuru, Kenya. This is the kind of industry urgently in need of development in Africa. The pyrethrum flowers grow well and Kenya is by far the greatest exporter in the world of this insecticide.

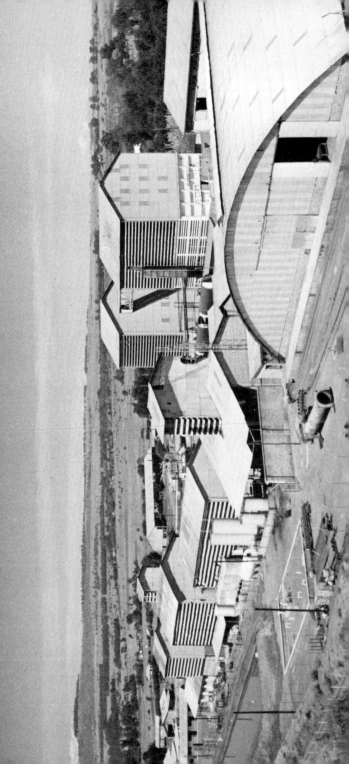

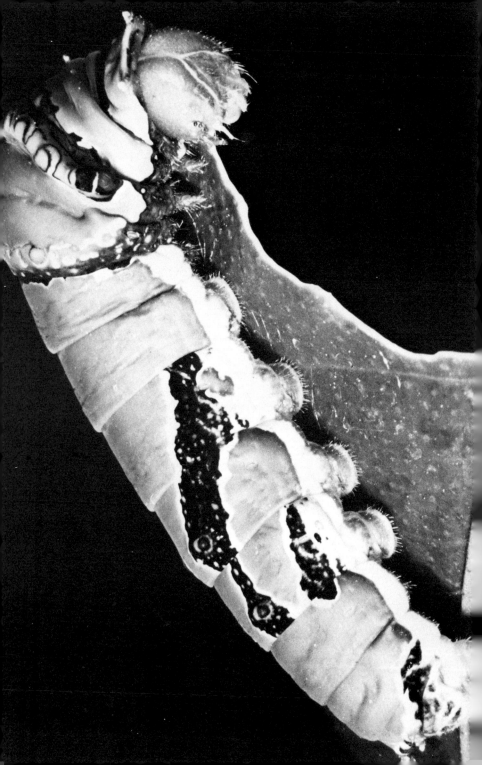

clearing the bush where the flies rest, and at killing the wild animals that act as reservoirs for the disease. None of these has succeeded completely (Glover, 1965). Insecticides have also been used, but one difficulty encountered is that the flies are on the whole rather rare (Glasgow, 1963) and it is thus not easy to eliminate them altogether. But whatever the merits of the schemes to eradicate the disease it is certain that there would today be far more cattle in Africa if it were not for trypanosomiasis. In view of the damage caused by cattle to the savanna grassland it may be that in the long run trypanosomiasis has slowed down the destruction of the environment. It would of course be desirable to develop a breed of cattle resistant to the disease and to limit its numbers by proper management of the feeding areas, but prospects for combining these two possibilities seem remote at present.

Numerous other diseases occur in African cattle, many of them transmitted by insects, ticks, and mites. These together with the scarcity of food of high nutrient value account for the poor quality of most of the cattle. But despite this the numbers of cattle continue to rise and there is little sign that a balance will be achieved between the numbers of cattle and the environment.

In both East and West Africa the nomads that look after and own cattle are characterized by their lack of respect for authority and their indifference to outside suggestions. Their cattle are of paramount importance and threats to their rights to graze cattle and to move as they please are resisted. In some areas the nomads have recently become cultivators, a step that is probably welcomed by most government administrators. It has for long been the custom of the Masai to take Kikuyu wives and this has often resulted in a more settled way of life. In West Africa it appears that the nomadic Fulani will become cultivators only when it is impossible for them to keep enough cattle for continued existence to be possible.

Nomadic pastoralists only kill their cattle for food as a last resort. Cattle that die naturally are eaten, and this probably produces a considerable quantity of meat, as the death rate in cattle is high. Many pastoralists also keep goats and sheep and these are more frequently killed for food. Milk is utilized whenever possible, but the production of milk depends upon a reasonable food supply for the cattle and on a relatively large herd if all members of the group

10 Larva of the butterfly, *Papilio demodocus*, feeding on *Citrus*. The young larvae feed on the new leaves and distort the growth pattern of young trees. The fully-grown larva (shown) is about 4 cm long.

are to receive some milk. Groups of nomadic Fulani depend almost entirely upon milk and milk products, either by consuming it themselves or by exchanging it for other foods from cultivators. The bleeding of cattle is common among the nomadic pastoralists, but it apparently occurs less frequently now than in the past. Leakey (1936) states that the blood of two cattle is required to provide a meal for about five Masai. The cattle are bled about once in every five or six weeks; more frequent bleeding would result in the cattle suffering. Allan (1965) calculates that a herd of 80 cattle (about 13 to 16 per person) would then be required to provide a family with one meal a day. Masai groups are commonly of three to eight families, averaging about five or six members to each family, and an average group owns about 300–700 cattle. These figures suggest that a nomadic group of Masai could subsist largely on blood obtained from their cattle, and this may indeed have been so until recently, but nowadays they probably depend to a large extent on the killing of smaller kinds of domesticated animals, including goats and chickens. Old reports of cattle owners cutting 'steaks' from living cattle seem doubtful.

As with cattle it appears that sheep spread into Africa from Asia and all the evidence suggests that they came in via Egypt and the Nile Valley. The domesticated sheep has been named *Ovis aries*, but its origin is uncertain. Sheep are best adapted to cool temperate grasslands and the existing tropical breeds are those that are better able to withstand drought and seasonal food shortage. Many pastoralists, including the Masai, keep flocks of sheep as well as cattle, but the social importance of sheep is not nearly so great as that of cattle. They are kept mainly for meat, and to a small extent for milk, skins, and hair. Wool-producing sheep do not flourish in the tropics, except at high elevations in East Africa. Owners of sheep allow them to breed freely and a typical flock may contain a large diversity of breeds. The growth rate of tropical African sheep is only about a quarter of that of sheep on temperate grassland (Williamson and Payne, 1965) and, like cattle, they are in general of poor quality. But quality is to some extent compensated for by quantity, and in many areas the sheep population is high and is continuing to expand to the detriment of the environment.

Domesticated goats are probably descendants of *Capra oegagrus* or of a related species, and they originated in mountainous areas of Asia. They are kept alongside cattle and sheep by most nomadic pastoralists, and are also common in villages, even in the forested regions of Africa. They have been allowed to breed freely and have become locally adapted to the climate and biotic conditions in the environments in which they live. Goats are essentially browsers and their ability to exploit almost all kinds of vegetation as well as a wide range of climates accounts for their abundance and distribution in Africa. Goats are kept mainly for meat and skins and in some areas, notably in Kikuyuland, they are remarkably productive. Since goats are browsers they are often destructive to forests, and in culti- vated areas they may initiate severe erosion of the soil on steep slopes by removing the vegetation. Government officials concerned with livestock are inclined to discourage the keeping of goats, but throughout tropical Africa they flourish and are commonly slaugh- tered for festive occasions or are used instead of money in exchange for other commodities.

Domesticated pigs appear to be hybrids between *Sus vittatus*, a wild pig of south-east Asia, and *Sus scrofa*, the European wild pig. They are rather uncommon in tropical Africa, probably because of the religious beliefs of the Muslims. Pigs feed on plant and animal material that could be referred to as refuse, and thus survive best in areas where there is considerable food wastage. Pigs produce large quantities of manure and the possibility of using this to enrich fish ponds in areas of protein shortage has been explored: it has been advocated that pig keeping and the development of fish ponds should proceed together. Pigs are kept mainly for their meat which seems to be more in demand in towns than in rural areas.

In most areas wild mammals are hunted and trapped. The range of traps used is a study in itself and there are some spectacular guns in use, some of which would gladden the heart of a museum curator. Besides the larger herbivorous species, almost all kinds of mammals, including rodents and monkeys, are esteemed, but there is much local and ethnic variation as to which kinds are eaten and which are not. Other terrestrial vertebrates, such as snakes and birds, are collected for food, and these, together with mammals, are probably important supplements to the protein-deficient diet of people in the forest region. But it seems strange that the hunting and trapping of birds has not reached the scale that it has in some other parts of the world, such as the Mediterranean region.

The main event in human ecology that has taken place in the last thousand years or so is the conversion of most of the population from hunting and gathering to cultivating and herding. During this time the negroids expanded in numbers and have almost eliminated the pygmies of the forest and the bushmen of the arid regions. The cultivators occupy the forest region and the more humid parts of the savanna while the pastoralists have occupied the more arid areas. A large but unknown proportion of the population of tropical Africa indulge in both activities, but in general the two ways of life are ecologically and geographically separated and have engendered a considerable amount of mutual distrust. The pastoralists probably stand to lose most in the long run as they are not favoured by national administrators, and the trend is for cultivation to increase at the expense of pastoralism. Both groups depend on products of low quality, the pastoralists on unproductive cattle and other domesticated animals, and the cultivators on root and cereal crops that in general are of low nutritional value. Both groups are also expanding in numbers and the fact that in tropical Africa there has been little sign of widespread famine (in contrast to some other tropical regions) is mainly because there is still adequate space. But as numbers increase the demand for space will become more acute and for continued survival the people will have to consolidate their plant and animal husbandry, and will have to use the land more efficiently than at present. Whether this will be possible remains to be seen.

CHAPTER 8

Food and Nutrition

The amount and quality of food required for a person to remain in normal health depends on age, sex, occupation, height, weight, and the climate in which the person lives. Because of these variables it is difficult to be precise about the normal requirements of food for an average person. The amount of food consumed should be sufficient to provide energy for normal activities, and it is suggested by nutritionists that a daily intake of below 2000 kcal is too little, while above 3000 kcal is too much. A considerable proportion of the people in the tropics probably exist on diets that yield less than 2000 kcal a day, but in tropical Africa it is likely that on the whole diets are adequate in terms of energy requirements. Many people in Europe and North America eat too much food for good health, as can be seen by the numerous advertisements for methods of losing weight, and by the bulging stomachs of middle-aged business men.

Assuming that there is enough food available the only additional requirement is that it should be well diversified so as to include an adequate amount of protein and a wide range of organic and inorganic materials which can be collectively called 'protective substances' (Stamp, 1965). These protective substances are required in small quantity and consist essentially of minerals and vitamins derived from food. The absence of one or more of these minerals or vitamins increases an individual's probability of suffering from a disease, which in essence is a disease caused by a deficiency in the diet.

There has been much talk of the problems created in Africa by what is called malnutrition. Malnutrition in this context almost always refers to a deficiency of protein in the diet, especially in growing children, but this is a restricted use of the term, as malnutrition refers to any form of suffering generated by a poor diet, including the eating of too much as well as too little food. Affluent Africans grow fat very quickly and they therefore suffer from malnutrition in much the same way as their European counterparts. But no one has paid much attention to this aspect of malnutrition in Africa; instead attention has been focused on nutritional problems created by diets that are deficient in protein or in protective substances.

Famine and starvation usually result from an inadequate supply of carbohydrate food. This occurs seasonally in some of the drier parts of Africa but at present cannot be considered a serious problem. Famines may well occur in the future, although exactly when we shall start to hear of widespread food shortage in Africa cannot be predicted as the rate of population growth is not known for most areas, neither is the capacity of the environment to produce more food. This chapter, then, is mainly about under-nourishment in the form of deficiencies in protein intake and of diets that lack adequate amounts of protective substances.

'Kwashiorkor' is a Ghanaian word which is said to mean 'red-headed boy'.[1] It has been adopted in the literature to describe a disease which results from a deficiency of protein in the diet. The hair of African children suffering from the disease often turns a golden red colour and this presumably explains why the word is used to describe protein malnutrition. Kwashiorkor resulting from insufficient intake of protein is prevalent in growing children, and also in lactating and pregnant women, but especially in small children who for a variety of reasons are unable to obtain sufficient quantities of breast milk from their mothers. In tropical Africa the disease is common and widespread in the area where cultivators grow staple crops that contain only small amounts of protein. This area includes the whole of the forest belt and the more humid savanna; that is, all of tropical Africa that is not pastoral. Within this area there are of course smaller areas, mainly on the coast or near large rivers and lakes where fish are available for food, where kwashiorkor is effectively absent. It is also rare among people that have sufficient money to buy a diversity of foods, but even among these people it can occur because of traditional food preferences.

Table 19 shows the protein content of some common foods

[1] Various other meanings are attributed to the word 'kwashiorkor' and it is apparent that the word has been picked up and used in different ways in different areas. It is not absolutely certain that the word is Ghanaian in origin.

expressed as a percentage of the dry and the fresh weight. As shown, cassava contains hardly any protein and the values for other root crops grown in tropical Africa, although not as low as for cassava, indicate that these are all deficient in protein. Maize contains more protein than most root crops and this together with the fact that in maize-growing areas there are usually livestock, suggests the savanna people are less likely to suffer from protein malnutrition than those in the forest region. I have included the values for spinach; many of the wild leaves that are gathered and used in sauces are probably of about the same value as spinach.

Kwashiorkor is caused by a chronic shortage of protein and a relative excess of carbohydrate in the diet. Many effects have been identified. Several enzymes and proteins may be deficient, the lipoprotein value is low, bone marrow activity is low, and there is a failure to produce enough haemoglobin, while in extreme cases the hair becomes golden, the skin pale, lesions appear on the body, the eyesight begins to fail, and the child refuses to feed. The disease is not difficult to cure and an adequate supply of milk can result in what appears to be a complete recovery within a very short time. There is however increasing evidence that there are long-term effects including heart disease in later life and mental retardation, and it is thus likely that severe kwashiorkor in childhood causes permanent damage. This is not astonishing as the disease tends to occur when growing babies are developing into small children, a most critical period both physically and mentally. The death rate among children suffering from kwashiorkor is difficult to estimate mainly because an individual suffering from the disease is much more prone to other diseases, particularly malaria, and death may result from the combined effects of several conditions occurring simultaneously. There is ample evidence that much child mortality in rural Africa is associated directly or indirectly with a diet that is deficient in protein. The effect of protein malnutrition on adults is less striking, and it is rarely in itself a killer, although it is believed to be responsible for lack of vigour, a failure to develop resistance to infectious diseases, and low mental abilities.

Kwashiorkor is not of course an infectious disease: it is the direct effect of a bad diet on individual health. Even in areas where carbohydrate staples form the main item of diet the disease could be reduced if there were not so many taboos and traditions about food. In some areas these discriminate against the children and the women, the people that are most likely to need an adequate diet. In September 1963 I attended a lecture at Kampala given by an eminent nutritionist. After outlining the causes of kwashiorkor he went on to deal with the sociological aspects of the disease among the Baganda, a group of people who subsist largely on a diet of protein-deficient bananas and whose children suffer severely from kwashiorkor. He pointed out that in Buganda the men get the meat and the children the gravy. Fish is not eaten much because of the bones. It is not the custom to spend much money on food and little is spent on the children. Milk is not regarded as a suitable drink, and children are sent away from home when one year old, as a living child is thought to be a danger to an unborn child. Another excuse for sending the children away is that it will help them to become 'independent'. The speaker emphasized that many people in Buganda do not understand the nutritional value of food or that food is converted into flesh, or that its quality is of importance to a growing child. I do not know how true all of these statements are, but there is probably some truth in most of them as similar attitudes have been described from many other parts of tropical Africa. It would certainly have been possible for some disagreement with the speaker if there had been people in the audience qualified to disagree. The lecture theatre was packed and the lecture was delivered in the heart of Africa at a well-known university famous for its medical school. And yet there was not one African in the audience. This incident possibly helps to explain the prevalence of kwashiorkor even in areas where people are relatively sophisticated: many Africans will not admit that there is such a condition and laugh nervously when the subject is raised. This is why so little is done to improve the nutrition of the children. A medical friend once told me that at a baby show in Uganda children with fair hair and puffed faces were given prizes as the best-looking babies. The children were suffering from kwashiorkor.

From what has been said so far it will be appreciated that kwashiorkor is as much a social problem as anything else, and its prevention will require more than simply providing the people in the carbohydrate belt with foods that contain protein. This aspect of the problem is well illustrated by Gerlach (1965) in his discussion of the sociology of nutrition among the Kigo of the Kenya coast. Kwashiorkor is not uncommon among the children but it is believed by the people to be caused by the breaking of a sexual taboo by the parents. The term 'chirwa' which means 'to do something forbidden' is used to describe the condition. Europeans have translated chirwa to mean protein malnutrition, but this is not what it means in Kigo. When the medical authorities ask to see children suffering from chirwa they are usually shown no one since the people do not like admitting that they have broken taboos. And then when European medical officers urge the people to give their children better food they are regarded by the Kigo as foolish and presumptuous because obviously one cannot remedy a broken taboo by eating certain foods. They believe instead that only traditional methods administered by specialists can be used to deal with chirwa. It is evident that even with the best intentions it would be difficult to remedy the frequency of kwashiorkor among these people.

But despite the above considerations much effort is being devoted to improving the nutritional quality of food in tropical Africa. Numerous suggestions have been put forward, a few have been implemented with varying results, but for the vast majority of people suffering from kwashiorkor the situation remains unchanged. In recent years attention has been focused on the use of vegetable proteins as a means of improving the quality of the diet. Some nutritionists argue that man needs animal protein and that proteins obtained from plants contain inadequate amounts of certain amino acids, notably lysine, but the possibility of producing such compounds synthetically and adding them to plant diets is now good, although the cost would be high. It does appear however that many people in the world never or hardly ever consume animal food. Protein can be extracted from leaves and according to Pirie (1966) it can be presented in a palatable form and could go a long way to reduce the present protein shortage in the humid tropics. Pirie acknowledges the social problem of people being resistant to change, but suggests that it is possible to change attitudes to food, citing as evidence for this the remarkable ability of food manufacturers to influence the habits of people by repeated advertising of their products. The numerous varieties of beans are rich in protein and increased production and consumption of these by the cultivators would also reduce protein malnutrition, provided plant protein is sufficient to take care of human needs. Kwashiorkor in tropical Africa could be reduced to negligible proportions simply by increasing the diversity of food crops grown so as to include plants known to be rich in protein, but there remains the difficulty of persuading people to eat what is good for them. Nutritionists doubting the efficacy of plant protein as a cure for kwashiorkor should bear in mind that the gorilla, a close relative of man, is entirely herbivorous, and shows no sign of protein malnutrition.

The development of fisheries and the increased use of fish in the diet is much favoured by outside experts, particularly by members of the Food and Agriculture Organization of the United Nations, as a means of reducing the prevalence of kwashiorkor in Africa and elsewhere in the tropics. It is pointed out that the fishery resources of Africa are under-exploited and that many of the methods of obtaining fish are inefficient and have continued unchanged for thousands of years. The last part of this statement is certainly true; and in addition Africa's marine fishing grounds are being increasingly exploited by boats from as far away as Korea and Japan. In Sierra Leone it is possible to buy fish obtained by Koreans just off the coast and yet the Sierra Leoneans themselves show little interest in developing their capacity to utilize the nearby resources, although there is of course much talk of doing this.

Between 1938 and 1961 the average rate of fish production in Africa increased by about 6 per cent per year. In 1960 tropical Africa produced about a million metric tons of fish, about half of it from marine fisheries on the West Coast and about half from fresh waters inland (Chapman, 1965). Fish production on the East Coast is small because of the unsuitable marine environment for fish, but research is being expanded to try and forecast how and when fish can be best obtained in this area. Before most of the African countries became independent there was fairly intensive research on both freshwater and marine fishery resources. This research was organized mainly on a regional basis. But after independence and with the development of nationalism these research organizations suffered severe set-backs and some have virtually ceased to exist as viable units. Various attempts have been made to revive them, chiefly by help from the specialized agencies of the United Nations and through bilateral aid from European countries. The development of nationalism has also reduced the activities of the local fishermen. Thus before independence Ghanaian fishermen moved freely with their canoes between the Congo and The Gambia, but this has now largely come to a halt as they are not allowed to cross territorial boundaries. (Several thousand Ghanaian fishermen were recently deported from Sierra Leone.) It would appear that dried and smoked fish was more freely available ten or so years ago than it is now. Efforts are now being directed towards encouraging each country to develop its own fishing fleet and to adopt modern methods of catching and processing the fish.

I have often heard experts express the view that the fishery resources off the African coast are virtually limitless, and that every effort should be made to exploit these resources. The resources are not of course limitless, and as more and more nations undertake long distance fishing trips there will be increased competition for the available fish and it will not be long before we hear cries that the African waters have been overfished, in much the same way as the waters around Europe and North America.

Africa is extremely rich in species of freshwater fish and there are numerous rivers and lakes that provide good fishing grounds. In 1961 it was estimated that tropical Africa produced between 10 and 20 per cent of the world's freshwater fish catch. Three areas are especially productive: the River Niger in Mali, the Lake Chad area, and the lakes of the eastern Congo, Rwanda, Burundi, Uganda, and Tanzania. The bulk of the fish caught belong to various species of *Tilapia*, members of the family Cichlidae that thrive in African freshwaters. Most of the fish caught are dried and smoked, but in some areas, notably at Lake George in Uganda, factories have been set up to freeze and package the fish. Outsiders observing the widespread occurrence of kwashiorkor in tropical Africa have advocated the development of fish ponds and fish farms. In the 1950s massive programmes to develop fish farming were initiated, particularly in the Congo where in quite a short time there were 100 000 individually owned ponds. In some ways these ponds created more problems than they solved. Water-borne diseases were introduced into areas where they had previously been absent, and malarial mosquitoes increased.[1] In addition many of the ponds received insufficient attention and the fish multiplied rapidly and never attained a good size. It was then discovered that many species of *Tilapia* would hybridize and that the resulting offspring were either predominantly or entirely males (Whitehead, 1960; Pruginin, 1965). This meant that ponds could be stocked with males only and since reproduction was impossible the fish attained a good size. Fish ponds, like all development projects, produce problems as well as helping to solve them. Many people have been quick to point out the value of fish ponds and *Tilapia* in tropical Africa, sometimes assuming that such projects will solve nutritional deficiencies by providing an abundance of animal protein. But again lurking behind these efforts is the seemingly insurmountable problem of persuading people to eat what is good for them.

Calcium, phosphorus, fluorine, and magnesium are needed by growing children for the growth and development of bones and teeth, and a deficiency of these minerals in the diet or in the drinking water results in the failure of the bones and teeth to grow properly and in decay of the teeth. Iron, phosphorus, and sulphur are important constituents of blood, liver, and muscle. A deficiency of iron often results in anaemia. The eating of small quantities of clay and earth by people, especially pregnant women, in parts of West Africa is probably an adaptation that makes good a deficiency of iron, and possibly also calcium. Sodium chloride (salt) is constantly lost from the body through sweating and urinating, and throughout tropical Africa salt is much in demand and is added to food in considerable amounts. Iodine deficiency, which results in goitre, is widespread in West Africa, mainly because the water is deficient in this substance. In Eastern Nigeria up to 40 per cent of the people suffer from goitre, and there is evidence that this high incidence may also be associated with the presence of a goitrogen in cassava, the staple food in the area (Ekpechi *et al.*, 1966).

Other minerals are needed in small quantities to maintain normal body metabolism. All are automatically acquired if the diet is diversified, but concentration of consumption on one or two staples can easily lead to deficiencies.

[1] There is of course no reason to worry about creating fish ponds in areas where malarial mosquitoes already occur, such as in fields of swamp rice.

Natural foods also contain organic compounds that are required by the body in even smaller quantities. These substances, the vitamins, are often destroyed during the cooking and processing of food, and their main source in a functional form is fresh fruit and vegetables. A deficiency in any of them results in poor growth in children. Vitamin A occurs in fish oils, liver, butter, cheese, and eggs, and also in fresh vegetables and tomatoes. The main source of vitamin A in tropical Africa is probably tomatoes and fish. A shortage of vitamin A results in poor growth in children and eye defects that impair vision. Several different vitamins are included in the B group. One of these, thiamine, occurs in meat, bread, beer, and the husk of rice. A shortage of thiamine can in extreme cases cause beri-beri, the occurrence of which is chiefly associated with a diet of milled rice. Beri-beri starts as a disease of the muscles, leading to paralysis, and eventually to heart failure. Ascorbic acid or vitamin C is derived from fresh fruit, especially citrus fruits. The widespread consumption of fresh oranges in the humid regions of tropical Africa probably provides sufficient quantities of vitamin C. A deficiency can lead to scurvy and, at least in areas where oranges abound, the presence of scurvy in the population is the result of an unexplained reluctance to eat fresh fruit. Vitamin D facilitates the deposition of calcium and phosphorus in bone and its absence leads to rickets. It is derived mainly from fish and its formation in the body is stimulated by ultra-violet rays received from sunlight. Rickets is a common disease among the cultivators of tropical Africa where fish is not available, and although it might be supposed that the tropics would provide an abundance of sunlight, ultra-violet radiation is not as intense as might be expected.

Mineral and vitamin deficiencies occur almost everywhere in tropical Africa and the cause is essentially lack of variety in the diet. The widespread use of wild plants as food goes some way to make up these deficiencies, but the plants are usually cooked which destroys some of the vitamins. There is an increasing tendency to use imported tinned foods as supplements to the diet, and even in rural villages there is often a store where tinned sardines, milk, and other cheap products may be bought. The use of these items, even on a small scale, probably reduces deficiency diseases to some extent.

Most people in tropical Africa who are no longer dependent on wild foods collect insects for food. The habit is especially well-developed among the cultivators of the forest region whose normal diet is deficient in protein, but it is uncertain whether insects are eaten because of their nutritional qualities. In some areas there is much ritual associated with the seasonal appearance of certain desirable species of insect. The eating of insects may in some ways be compared with the European tendency to eat marine molluscs and crustaceans. The aversion to insects as human food among Europeans is probably based on nothing more than custom and prejudice: insects are indeed good to eat and some taste as good as the best lobster or crab.

The literature on insects in the diet of man is scattered through numerous books and journals devoted to travel, ethnology, geography, medicine, and biology, but fortunately much of what has been published has been abstracted and summarized by Bodenheimer (1951). In Africa, the main groups of insects utilized are members of the Orthoptera (grasshoppers), Isoptera (termites), Coleoptera (beetles), and Lepidoptera (moths, but only the larvae). The species utilized within these groups are those that are locally or seasonally abundant. Examples are locusts and other Orthoptera which at times can be extremely abundant, the winged reproductives of termites which occur in immense numbers with the onset of the rains, and the gregarious larvae of moths, particularly members of the Saturniidae. As with some other foods there are often ceremonies and beliefs as well as discriminatory taboos built into the collecting and eating of species that are locally important. Thus almost everywhere certain segments of the community are forbidden to eat insect delicacies: sometimes the women are not allowed to eat them, sometimes the children, sometimes sick people, pregnant women, and so on. It appears that some insects are held in high esteem and are therefore reserved by custom for the more important and senior members of the community, and if someone is found eating insects that are by custom taboo there may be unpleasant consequences for that person.

Throughout tropical Africa there are many species of termites, some confined to savanna, others to forest. The larger species are much favoured as food and in many areas of East Africa the termite mounds are owned and protected by individual families. Anyone caught collecting termites from a privately owned mound is likely to be regarded as a thief. The winged reproductives leave the mounds in immense numbers with the first heavy rainfall that marks the onset of the wet season, and a wide variety of traps is used to catch them as they emerge. Termite bodies are soft and fat and they are either eaten raw or lightly fried in their own fat. Winged termites shed their wings soon after leaving the mound and this facilitates dealing with them as food. Most species are attracted to lights and lights are utilized as a means of collecting them. Each mound contains one or more queens which are large and very fat, and probably highly nutritious as they are full of eggs. Owners of mounds would probably hesitate to destroy the colony by taking the queen, but queens are taken from mounds located away from villages where there appears to be no question of ownership. The queens are regarded as a delicacy and eating them is often reserved for a special occasion. Bodenheimer (1951) reports that in some areas of the Congo the entire village may sleep by day in order to spend the night collecting termites. In eastern Uganda winged termites are induced to leave the mound by beating the nearby ground with sticks. This apparently simulates heavy rainfall and the termites frequently respond by swarming out as if after a shower of rain. The worker and the soldier termites, being much smaller and less fat, are not widely sought after as food, but in some areas, notably in parts of the Congo, the mounds are opened up by children who place leaves in the chambers which the soldiers bite. The leaves are then withdrawn with the termites attached. In some areas there is a considerable trade in termites. They are dried in the sun, wrapped in leaves, and transported to markets, sometimes being sent long distances. In many East African towns and villages it is possible to buy sun-dried termites at the local market at the right season of the year.

When locusts arrive in dense swarms they are usually regarded as pests but to some people they are a welcome sight. The three species that are especially injurious to crops (Chapter 6) are esteemed by many people as food. They are usually fried, but there are numerous other recipes, including pounding them up and adding the mixture to sauces. They taste good and resemble shrimps in flavour. Although cultivators may suffer enormously from a locust plague they make the most of the locusts by catching as many as possible and eating them. Other members of the Orthoptera are also eaten, particularly the long-horned bush cricket, *Homorocoryphus nitidulus*, which in East Africa occurs in immense swarms with the onset of the rains. It flies at night and is attracted to lights where it can be collected easily. The females in particular are very fat, probably because the insect is a long-distance migrant. In Uganda the species is known as 'nsenene' and the Abdim's stork which tends to follow the swarms is known as the 'nsenene bird'. Flights of these birds herald the arrival of nsenene and in some areas a special watch is kept for them. There are many local customs associated with the collecting and eating of nsenene. One dictates that a male and a female must always be released from among those collected so as to make sure that numbers can be replenished by breeding. The females of *Homorocoryphus nitidulus* have a long ovipositor and it is widely believed that this is the penis of the male; thus the two sexes are differentiated but the females are thought to be males, and vice versa. There are several distinct colour forms, some of them rare; the Luganda name for one of these forms means that if such a form is found there should be many nsenene within a limited period, an observation that is biologically sound as the appearance of a form that occurs naturally at a frequency of one in five thousand or so may be taken to indicate that the species is common in the area. The introduction of powerful electric street lights into towns in East Africa has revolutionized nsenene collecting as the insects are attracted in vast numbers to these lights. At Kampala in Uganda the streets may be completely blocked to traffic by people who come in from rural areas to collect nsenene.

Crickets that live in the ground are obtained by digging for them. At dusk many species sing loudly from their burrows and they are thus located and dug up. A large and fat species, *Brachytrypes membranaceus*, is regarded as a particular delicacy and is dug up from compounds where it is apt to be destructive to root crops.

The larvae of many of the larger beetles are sought after and eaten. They are usually roasted and eaten whole, except for the head. Beetles are not as important as termites and grasshoppers in the diet as there are few really common species, and even these do not occur

11 *Lantana camara*, an abundant weed introduced into Africa from tropical America. Efforts are being made to control the spread of the weed by introducing insects that feed on it.

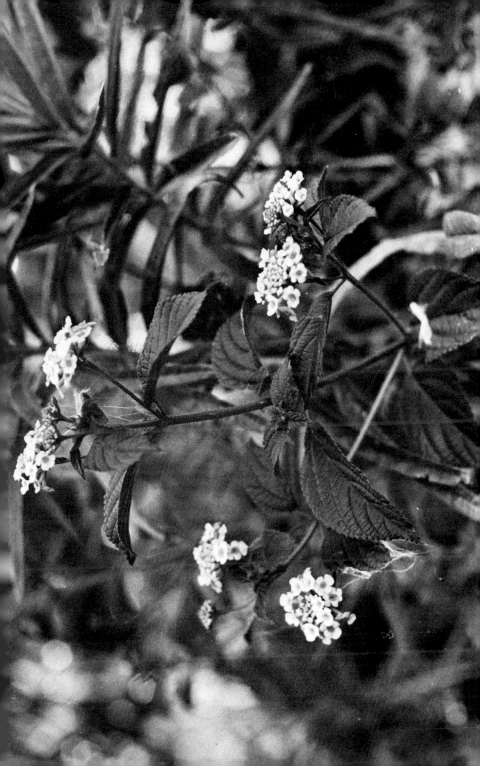

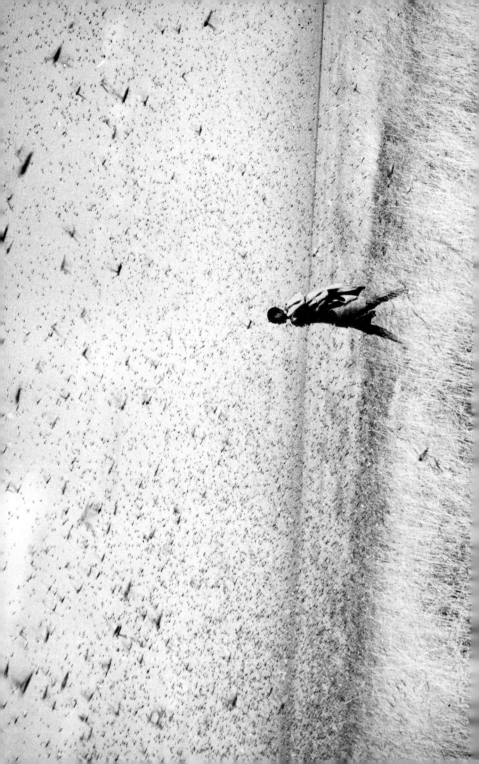

in large swarms. Moth larvae are collected and roasted, and may often be bought in the markets. The East African lakes support immense populations of the larvae of aquatic flies. The adults of some of these species, particularly members of the genus *Chaoborus*, emerge periodically in great numbers often in association with the phases of the moon. Great clouds of flies may drift ashore from the lake. They are collected by whirling baskets attached to long handles into the swarm and when the basket is full of flies they are squashed and dried in the sun. Lakefly cakes are possibly an important source of protein in Uganda and elsewhere in East Africa.

Almost everywhere in Africa honey is much sought after and many varieties of beehive have been invented. The introduction of *Eucalyptus* trees from Australia and their establishment in swamps, to provide drainage as part of the programme to control mosquitoes, has produced excellent conditions for apiculture as the flowers of these trees are attractive to bees and the resulting honey is of high quality. The nests of wild bees are also exploited, and besides the honey, bee larvae are also collected for food. The exploitation of bees for their honey occurs throughout the world and the cultural aspects of honey-getting and the domestication of bees is a subject in itself.

Among numerous groups of people that include insects in their diet are the Baganda who live around the northern shore of Lake Victoria in Uganda. But the Baganda are better known for their preoccupation with the cultivation and preparation of bananas as their main item of food. There are banana gardens everywhere and the staple food of the rural people consists of steamed cooking bananas (or plantains), especially varieties that are known locally as matoke (or matooke). In southern Uganda bananas grow well and require little attention, and they are relatively free of pests and diseases. Most people grow enough to feed themselves, but considerable quantities are sent to towns and marketed. A common sight in the region is a taxi carrying an enormous quantity of bananas on the roof; this probably represents a surplus that a family is sending to market for sale.

The climate of southern Uganda is rather uniform all the year round, rain falling in every month of the year, and there is rarely a shortage of food. Adults take one or more large meals of matoke each day usually accompanied by a variety of side dishes which are

12 A swarm of desert locusts in Ethiopia, September 1958. These insects may destroy the crops of millions of people living in the drier areas of Africa.

mainly sauces. Rutishauser (1962) has given a detailed description of the preparation of matoke and the side dishes. There is a considerable amount of ritual associated with the preparation of the meal. Thus when considered ripe (and this in itself may involve considerable discussion) the banana stem is carefully cut down and the leaves removed, but these leaves are not used for wrapping the food; instead fresh leaves are cut from an adjacent tree. The leaves in which the matoke is to be wrapped are cut with a special hooked knife attached to a rod, the use of the correct knife being most important. An elephant grass stem may not be used for the rod as this will bring hail to the banana garden. Banana leaves are used not only to wrap the food but also as aprons and to cover the floor. Cleanliness is regarded as most important and there is frequent hand-washing by the women preparing the meal. Each banana is skinned with a special knife and when enough have been prepared the cooking pot is lined with banana leaves, water is added, and a tied bundle of matoke, together with any additional small bundles of other items, is placed in the pot. The first cooking takes between one and one and a half hours, the matoke is then removed and kneaded, and then cooked for a further one to two hours. The entire operation from the collection of the bananas to the eating of the meal takes between three and a quarter and five and a quarter hours, which, considering the operation is performed daily, is remarkably time-consuming. The few other staples are prepared in a similar way, often being cooked with the matoke. Special banana leaves are used for packaging the sauces which are to become side dishes. Ground-nuts form the basis of many sauces, and these must be of considerable nutritional importance. A wide variety of green leaves, including those of wild plants, is used, and mushrooms gathered from near termite mounds are regarded as a most acceptable addition. Small tomatoes, beans, eggs, fish, and meat are incorporated into the sauces whenever available, and fried grasshoppers and termites are eaten as snacks between the main meals. There is usually plenty to eat, but the food is deficient in protein, which perhaps is not especially important for the adults, but often results in conspicuous malnutrition in the children.

Similar meals based on bananas or on other staples are prepared throughout rural Africa where subsistence crops are grown. Almost all of the staples have been introduced into Africa from other tropical regions of the world and yet there is much ceremony attached to the way the crops are harvested and prepared for eating. The method of propagating cassava by planting cut stems varies in different groups of people, each group using a specific method and no other. These methods have been developed in relatively recent times and yet they have the appearance of ancient traditions.

Throughout tropical Africa there are groups of people that exploit a local source of food which in other areas is ignored. An example of this is the capture of clawed toads, *Xenopus* sp., in the lakes of Kigezi, Uganda. The toads are dried in the sun and eaten whole and the exploitation is confined to a small area where the main foods are cultivated crops. The nutrient qualities of these toads are not known, but since they are not cooked and are presumably rich in protein, they probably provide an important source of essential nutrients to people whose main diet is root crops and maize. Another example is the collection and local marketing of large land snails of the family Achatinidae. These snails are common in tropical Africa, but there are vast areas where they are not utilized for food. In the Congo, Ghana, and in some other countries in West Africa, they are collected and eaten, but east of Uganda they are ignored. They are large and rich in protein and thus contribute substantially to the nutrition of people that eat them.

The clam, *Egeria radiata*, has been collected from the lower Volta River for centuries, judging by the deposits of shells along the banks of the river. It occurs also in the lower reaches of other West African rivers, including the Sanaga in Cameroon. The exploitation of these clams has been described by Lawson (1963) and Pople (1966). *Egeria radiata* is believed to be a relatively recent colonist of fresh water as it belongs to a predominantly marine group and it has not penetrated far up the West African rivers. The collection and marketing of these clams is entirely in the hands of the women, between one and two thousand being involved in the enterprise on the Volta. About 4000–7000 metric tons of clams are collected each year and these yield about 50 tons of protein. The young clams are collected at the beginning of the dry season in December and January and are transported alive to 'farms' located upstream. The farms are specially prepared sections of shallow water which are stocked with clams at a density of about 1560 m². At the end of the dry season the clams are collected from the farms and are prepared for sale in the market. With the construction of the Volta Dam at Akosombo the flow of the river has been altered and regulated and this is causing a change in the distribution and abundance of the clams. The clam populations in the Sanaga River are subject to marked fluctuations in size which have not been explained, but the women who collect the clams do not at the present stock upstream farms in the way that is customary on the Volta. There are occasionally good years for clams in the Sanaga, and Pople (1966) reports that at the end of a good season men have stopped the women from going to the market because they become too rich and get ideas above their station. The flesh of the clams is incorporated into the normal diet of the people living near these rivers and there is no doubt that it is an important source of animal protein.

For many years the governments and people of tropical African nations have received advice from others as to how nutrition can be improved. Much effort on the part of the Food and Agriculture Organization of the United Nations is devoted to the problem of malnutrition, and many bilateral aid projects set out specifically to do the same job. Charitable organizations in Europe and America frequently draw attention to malnutrition in Africa as a means of raising funds. Curiously enough some individuals have also felt obliged to join in the cry for improved nutrition. Pamphlets are circulated urging the governments and people to take action to improve the state of nutrition. Some years ago when I was working in Sierra Leone I received a copy of the following suggestion. It was addressed to the 'Premiers of all countries' and was signed by John J. Light, 414 South Kaley, South Bend, Indiana, U.S.A. Part of the pamphlet is headed 'Answer to food shortage' and it goes on to say,

A California Institute of Technology scientist and nutritionist Dr. Henry Borsock, described how the calcium of the white cliffs of Dover was used in England in World War II to feed children in place of milk because there was not enough milk. Such chalk cliffs (made of the bones of ancient sea animals) are available all over the world, and should be used to prevent starvation. I hope you can put your scientists and industry to work immediately to utilize this source of calcium.

CHAPTER 9

Human Diseases

For many years it has been known that viruses may cause tumours in mammals other than man and until recently it appeared that man was inexplicably different in this respect. But the discovery by Burkitt (1958) of a cancer affecting the jaws of African children and the subsequent mapping of its distribution in tropical Africa, during which it was shown to be most frequent in high rainfall and high temperature areas, provided the possibility that a human cancer had been discovered that was caused by a virus, possibly transmitted by an insect vector. In some areas of Africa more than half the cases of cancer in children can be attributed to the Burkitt tumour, or Burkitt's lymphoma as it is often called (Ngu, 1967). Its geographical distribution and high relative frequency among children, together with its occurrence among adults who have recently arrived in an area where it is prevalent and its absence in resident adults, suggest that immunity to the disease can be acquired, and this again suggests a virus as the causal agent. Burkitt's lymphoma has now been found in other parts of the tropics and also in some temperate areas, and viruses have been isolated from the tumour, but whether these cause the tumour has not yet been established. Much effort has been devoted to a search for an insect vector (Haddow, 1963; Wright *et al.*, 1967; Williams, 1967), but thus far a possible vector has remained elusive. The lymphoma tends to occur most frequently in children living in settlements near permanent water and in the vicinity of dense vegetation, an environment much favoured by numerous species of mosquitoes, and after an intensive survey Goma (1965) concludes that 'the results do not conflict with the view that Burkitt's lymphoma syndrome may be caused by a mosquito-borne virus'. Besides the bones of the face the lymphoma may affect other parts of the body, including the abdomen, limb bones, and central nervous system. Patients suffering from the lymphoma are treated with drugs and a considerable degree of success is reported, which is probably not unrelated to an immunity response developing at the same time (Ngu, 1967).

Burkitt's contribution was to correlate the occurrence of the lymphoma with ecological and geographical features of the environment. The first step therefore was to map the distribution of the disease and to interpret the map in terms of geography and ecology. The implications of the results are considerable as for the first time in man there is the strong suggestion of a cancer caused by an insect-borne virus. Confirmation of this would presumably change the direction of much of the cancer research that is going on today.

I have started this chapter on human diseases with a summary of Burkitt's lymphoma because it indicates that not all medical effort in Africa is devoted to preventive measures and cures. The results of such research as this are appreciated throughout the world, especially in regard to possible cures for other lymphomas, and it may now be only a matter of time before the virus and its vectors are discovered.

Human diseases may be divided into two categories: those that are inherited, and those that are acquired by contact with some feature in the environment, frequently another organism. Much is known about the inheritance of disease in European populations (Stern, 1960; Clarke, 1970), but with a few exceptions, notably the sickle cell trait (discussed in Chapter 10), the subject has been neglected in tropical Africa, possibly because of the overwhelming complexity of diseases caused by the environment which seem to demand more immediate attention than those that are inherited. Thus in Britain haemophilia, an inherited sex-linked trait that results in a failure of the blood to coagulate properly, occurs at a rate of two or three per 100 000 of the population, and Christmas disease, which has similar effects, occurs at a frequency of about one-tenth of that of haemophilia. Both are therefore rare diseases and their frequency in the population may not be much above the theoretical mutation rate. Both diseases have been reported only rarely from Africa, but it seems that if a search is made the diseases are found, as in Kenya where Christmas disease is possibly more frequent than haemophilia (Forbes et al., 1966). It would appear that better facilities for diagnosis would show that these two diseases are more common in Africa than is commonly supposed, but

Forbes *et al.* mention the possibility that the widespread practice of ritual circumcision of males (who because the trait is sex-linked are more likely to have the disease) results in early death through haemorrhage if the blood is unable to coagulate.

Most of the diseases caused by the environment are the results of infections by viruses, funguses, bacteria, and Protozoa, while some are caused by metazoans which are often collectively referred to as 'worms', a term that covers a variety of different organisms. Many of these diseases are transmitted by insects, particularly Diptera, which because of their mode of feeding, injecting saliva and then sucking liquid food through the proboscis, provide the kind of mechanism that facilitates the transmission of disease. All of such diseases can be described as infectious. But there are other infectious diseases, notably cholera and typhoid, that are not transmitted by other organisms, but are water- or air-borne. Young children in particular are prone to infectious diseases and often after suffering from a specific disease develop an immunity such that they do not suffer again in later life, or at least do not suffer so badly. Virus diseases, such as measles, usually result in immunity to later infection, and immunity to diseases caused by Protozoa, such as malaria, also occurs. The impact of disease is far more devastating among populations suffering from one or more forms of malnutrition, and especially in the forest region of Africa malnutrition resulting from protein deficiency undoubtedly favours the spread and intensity of some of the common diseases. Many people who have studied diseases in tropical Africa have found it impossible to diagnose the exact cause of morbidity or mortality as in nearly all cases more than one disease is involved and the effects are often intimately associated with malnutrition.

The mapping of the distribution of diseases (sometimes called medical geography) and the association of the observed distributions with ecological features of the environment, including both biotic and climatic factors, provides the basis of programmes that aim at preventing diseases (Stamp, 1965). It might be added that consideration should also be given to changes in the environment brought about by man's actions. These include not only the development of cultivation, but also special projects such as the building of large reservoirs and small fish ponds. The rate of increase of the human population is also of great importance in this regard. All diseases thrive better at high population densities, but especially diseases that are transmitted from one person to another. An increase in abundance of disease vectors and in the frequency with which the disease occurs have been repeatedly noted whenever human populations rise without a corresponding expansion of medical facilities. This phenomenon is not of course confined to man: the predators, parasites, and diseases of all animals and plants tend to be relatively more abundant and more effective when the density of the prey or host is high than when it is low.

In man the transmission of disease is further complicated by international and intercontinental movements. This is why there are international regulations that require vaccinations and inoculations against some of the more dangerous of the world diseases, such as smallpox, cholera, and yellow fever. The recent outbreak of cholera in West Africa was almost certainly facilitated by the movement of people by aircraft from one country to another before it was realized that steps had to be taken to prevent people from travelling who had not been inoculated.

Other animals can be infected with human diseases. In Sierra Leone chimpanzees sometimes feed at refuse heaps around villages and as a result their teeth have become infected by eating contaminated food thrown out by people (Jones and Cave, 1960).

Outsiders repeatedly express concern about the prevalence of disease among the population of Africa and much effort has been devoted to preventive measures and cures. Unfortunately many of the efforts are of short-term duration and the result, especially in remote rural areas, is not only that the population increases, but also that the development of natural immunity is prevented or reduced such that when the people are left to their own devices again they suffer even more.

There are two additional problems. First, the use of drugs, vaccines, and antibiotics is rendered useless unless people can improve their own sanitary conditions. No progress will be made with the eradication of infectious disease unless the habits of the people can be changed. Katz and Koprowski (1967), in what they call a realistic approach to the eradication of disease, offer the following comment:

As improvement in man's sanitary environment is mainly responsible for progress in the control of contagious disease, so man's resistance to change of his habits and customs presents the single obstacle which slows down this progress. This principle applies to all peoples and all countries. It is as difficult to persuade man to use the privy as to stop smoking or to have sexual intercourse with contraceptives, for this involves breaking down his 'natural habits'.

Secondly, the conspicuous success of the use of antibiotics to cure disease is not without its difficulties. The problem is that the disease organism, like all other organisms, possesses the capacity for genetic change and evolution. The repeated use of antibiotics such as penicillin has resulted in the evolution of resistant strains of some bacteria. Not all antibiotics have thus far stimulated the evolution of resistant strains of the disease organism they are meant to kill, but it may only be a matter of time before they do, and then we shall be faced with new strains of some diseases, which, in turn, will promote further research to find new antibiotics. The process has no obvious end to it, but at the moment there is no other possibility except to continue along the same lines as before.

The main point that emerges in Chapter 6 is that in Africa insects are by far the most important threat to agriculture. Precisely the same situation exists for human diseases: insects are the greatest hazard to human health. Many of the common diseases in Africa are transmitted by insects either by their biting behaviour or by incidental contamination of food with bacteria. The ecology of human disease in Africa is, more closely than in most other places, correlated with the ecology of insects, and of the insects the Diptera stand out as being the most important source of infection.

Mosquitoes are members of the dipterous family Culicidae. In 1877 it was demonstrated for the first time that a human parasite, *Wuchereria bancrofti*, which causes filariasis, developed in a mosquito, and since that date it has been discovered that many other organisms causing human diseases undergo part of their development in mosquitoes. Transmission of the disease organism occurs when an infected mosquito bites a man (or other vertebrate) in order to take a meal of blood which is required for the mosquito to reproduce. Knowledge of mosquito-borne diseases has increased rapidly since the initial discovery was made, and today more than a thousand scientific papers are published a year on mosquitoes and mosquito-borne diseases (Mattingly, 1969). Most people think of mosquitoes as flies that transmit malaria, but they also transmit viruses, including those that cause yellow fever, and it is now thought that the prevention and eradication of many of the common tropical diseases can only be brought about by the application of control measures developed after a thorough understanding of the ecology of mosquitoes. Not all of the numerous species of mosquitoes transmit diseases. Indeed it is only a relatively narrow spectrum of mosquito species that is involved in the transmission of human diseases. Even within a species of mosquito there may be genetic strains that are incapable of sustaining a particular parasite.

Much of the effort devoted to the eradication of mosquito-borne diseases has been expended towards the destruction of mosquitoes either directly with insecticides or indirectly by draining the swampy places in which they breed. The possibility of controlling mosquito populations by genetic means has recently come into prominence. The methods being developed involve the sterilization of one sex by radiation and the release of substantial numbers into natural populations, and also the breeding of strains in which the sex ratio is significantly distorted. These techniques are likely to be of increasing importance in the future, especially as mosquitoes, like some other insects, have evolved strains that are resistant to insecticides. Many development projects in tropical Africa have resulted in the creation of new breeding places for mosquitoes. Thus swamps are drained to destroy mosquitoes but within the same area fish ponds are started which provide ideal habitats for the breeding mosquitoes. Some areas that have been cleared of one species of mosquito by the use of insecticides have been invaded by another species (Gillies and Smith, 1960).

The eggs of mosquitoes are laid in or near water. The eggs of some species can withstand months of desiccation while those of others must hatch within a short period or they perish. Different species of mosquitoes lay their eggs in different sites and the majority of species utilize the fresh water of ponds, swamps, and the numerous puddles that form in vegetation after rain. Interspecific differences in the sites used for egg-laying have been studied by placing small containers filled with water in a variety of positions in habitats utilized by mosquitoes. These containers are made of bamboo and provide a similar niche to that used by the numerous species that lay their eggs in water that has accumulated in holes in trees. The preference of different species can be deduced by scoring the frequency at which larvae appear in bamboo containers placed at different sites, especially at different levels in a forest (Corbet, 1964). The clearance of swamps as a means of reducing mosquito populations can result in a change in the diversity of species and can even lead to an overall increase in numbers (Goma, 1961). This is because clearing a swamp can leave numerous small bodies of water which are more favoured by some species than the rather enclosed water of a natural swamp. It follows from this that man-made containers, such as tins, abandoned motor car tyres, and similar products of civilization that are left scattered around the countryside, will provide excellent sites for the breeding of mosquitoes as soon as they begin to hold water. Empty coconut shells, which are such a feature of the coastal area of West Africa, provide similar sites, as do the empty shells of achatinid snails which have been thrown away by people who have collected the snails for food.

The larvae of mosquitoes tend to occur at high densities in relatively small volumes of water, the density achieved being determined in part by the organic matter in the container or body of water. Larval growth is extremely rapid and in some species the pupal stage lasts only a day or two. These life history characteristics enable a rapid increase in population size within a short time.

Many adult mosquitoes are crepuscular or nocturnal, but some are active during the day. The time of flight, the conditions under which flight will occur, and the habitats of the adults are characteristic of the species. Many tropical species undergo seasonal changes in numbers that in one way or another are associated with the alternation of wet and dry seasons. In general mosquitoes are more numerous in the wet season, but there are striking exceptions, as instanced by the sudden appearance of mosquitoes in houses during dry weather. It is known that wind speed and direction can modify the abundance of mosquitoes locally, and it appears that many species will drift on air currents for quite long distances.

Most species of mosquitoes feed as adults on the blood of terrestrial vertebrates, and a few species have been observed feeding on invertebrates. A few species do not feed on blood. The time of feeding and the kind of animal from which the blood is obtained vary not only with the species of mosquito, but also with different strains of a species and with the environment (Mattingly, 1969). The Protozoa that cause malaria and the viruses that cause a variety of diseases all develop to a certain degree in the mosquito vector. Without this development it appears that the successful transmission of the pathogen is impossible. The pathogen is transmitted from one host to another as the mosquito bites. There is no evidence that the pathogen harms the mosquito, but its survival is dependent on passing part of its life cycle in the mosquito. Since each species of mosquito tends to feed on the blood of a relatively narrow range of hosts it follows that the rate of transmission of the pathogen is dependent on the density of the host, and this is why diseases like malaria and yellow fever are potentially a greater threat in densely populated than in sparsely populated areas.

Although most people think of malaria as a specific disease, it is in reality a word applied to a wide range of diseases of warm-blooded vertebrates that are caused by Protozoa parasitizing the red blood cells. All forms of malaria appear to be transmitted by mosquitoes; no other vector is incriminated. Malarial parasites are collectively referred to as Haemosporidia, the classification and bionomics of which have been monographed by Garnham (1966). It has become the custom to restrict the term malaria to diseases caused by *Plasmodium*, four different species of which cause four different types of malaria in man. There are numerous accounts of the clinical and biological effects of malaria (Smyth (1962) provides a useful introduction to the subject), but the disease is characterized by a high fever which if not treated can rapidly cause death. *Plasmodium* parasites enter *Anopheles* mosquitoes when the mosquitoes bite an infected person. They then undergo development and a form of reproduction in the stomach of the mosquito before moving to the salivary gland from which they are transmitted to a person when the mosquito bites again. The fever develops quickly and in severe cases high fevers alternate with shivering fits, the periodicity of which varies with the species of *Plasmodium*.

Malaria was until recently the most widespread disease in the world, but it has been replaced by filariasis (Mattingly, 1969), a disease that is currently increasing because of inadequate sanitation which provides a favourable environment for its vector, the mosquito, *Culex pipiens fatigans*. Malarial infections respond quickly to drugs that act as a poison to the parasites in the red blood cells, and provided drugs are available there is no reason why a person should die of the disease. Malaria occurs throughout tropical Africa and efforts at control are mainly directed towards eradicating mosquitoes with insecticides. Eradication of malaria in an area has usually resulted in an increase in the population size and its attendant problems; moreover when eradication programmes have come to an end the disease can quickly return and the death rate can rise again. This pattern of events has been described for both East and West Africa (Pringle, 1966, 1969; McGregor, 1960). There is very little evidence that fluctuations in the intensity of malaria alter the birth rate of people.

Children who are exposed to malaria and recover develop a considerable degree of immunity to the disease in later life. This immediately raises the problem as to whether treatment of malaria with drugs is desirable in rural communities where the availability of such drugs in later life is uncertain. The immunological aspects of malaria have been examined in The Gambia by I. A. McGregor and his team from both the sociological and the biochemical point of view. Children exposed to malaria who receive no treatment elaborate antibodies, while those that are treated do not elaborate antibodies, and Voller and Wilson (1964) conclude that frequent infection is necessary to maintain immunity. Gambian women protected with doses of chloroquine (an anti-malarial drug) for two years showed a fall in gamma-globulin (serum protein) levels, but women that had not been protected showed no change in gamma-globulin level (Gilles and McGregor, 1961). But the women that were protected still maintained higher values of gamma-globulin than Europeans in the same area, despite their freedom from malaria for two years, and it is likely that other factors, both genetic and environmental, are involved. Poor nutrition and infections with other diseases might be the reason why higher gamma-globulin levels were maintained in these women. The capacity to develop immunity after infection with malaria (and with other diseases) varies with the individual, and it seems probable that there is a genetic component to the ability to produce an immunity response.

Individuals heterozygous for the sickle cell gene (Chapter 10) have considerable inherited resistance to malaria caused by *Plasmodium falciparum*. This is the commonest form of malaria in tropical Africa. The distribution and frequency of the sickle cell gene in human populations is correlated with the intensity of malaria. Several other inherited abnormal haemoglobins in man appear to be distributed and to occur at frequencies that suggest that individuals possessing the trait are resistant to various forms of malaria.

In many areas of Africa malaria, together with malnutrition, accounts for the widespread morbidity and high mortality among the people, especially among the children. It is known how both conditions can be prevented and eradicated, but what is not known is the consequence of eradication on the rate of growth of the human population.

Mosquitoes are also the vectors of other diseases. About eighty different kinds of viruses are known to be transmitted by mosquitoes, and more than half of these can infect man (Mattingly, 1969). Among these viruses are a few that cause the most killing of all the diseases that affect man. Viruses transmitted by arthropods (to which mosquitoes and all other insects belong) are known as arboviruses. The viruses multiply in the stomach of the vector and spread to other tissues, in mosquitoes especially to the salivary glands and the nervous system. When the mosquito bites a vertebrate host the virus is transmitted and multiplies extremely rapidly such that there is often a high concentration of the virus in the blood within a day or two. Many viruses introduced into the human body spread to almost all tissues, but some are associated with a particular tissue, notably those that cause encephalitis which results in severe and often permanent damage to the brain. The disease known as dengue is caused by several different and apparently unrelated viruses that in man produce similar symptoms, especially backache. The yellow fever virus is associated with the organs of the body, but especially with the liver.

The identification and isolation of arboviruses involves knowledge of both the vectors and the host. Such work was initiated in 1936 by what was then the Yellow Fever Research Institute at Entebbe in Uganda. This later became the East African Virus Research Institute and in the twenty-six years ending in December 1963 many arboviruses were isolated, thirteen of them for the first time (Woodall, 1964). The Institute also discovered additional mosquito species as vectors of yellow fever, and established that *Anopheles* mosquitoes (the usual vectors of malaria) are vectors of the virus that causes o'nyong nyong. It is beginning to become apparent that insects and other arthropods can potentially transmit a wide variety of viruses to man and other animals, but that only a relatively small number of them are likely to generate epidemics of disease.

Infection with a virus disease is often fatal, death taking place quickly, but some diseases caused by viruses, including o'nyong nyong, although extremely unpleasant, are rarely killers. Virus infections usually result in the elaboration of antibodies such that if the person survives subsequent infection is unusual.

The arbovirus causing yellow fever is transmitted by the mosquito, *Aedes aegypti*, and other species of the same genus. The disease originated in West Africa and was transmitted to the Americas by the slave trade. Inoculation against the disease is successful and evidence of inoculation is required from international travellers throughout the world. In 1960–2 a yellow fever epidemic in Ethiopia affected 200 000 people, killing 30 000 of them (Mattingly, 1969). This epidemic represents the easternmost extension of the disease and much interest has been aroused as it brought the disease much closer to the teeming millions of people in tropical Asia, a region that has thus far been unaffected. The introduction of the disease into India would undoubtedly have conspicuous results. A death from yellow fever was recorded in Uganda in 1964 and this prompted a careful search for the possible vector and the primate host of the virus (Haddow, 1965; Simpson *et al.*, 1965). The casualty from the disease came from a particular part of Uganda where monkeys are common and there was no evidence that he had travelled anywhere else. Yellow fever virus identical to that obtained from the casualty was found in *Aedes africanus* mosquitoes in the area, and one red-tailed monkey obtained near the victim's home showed a high level of antibody indicating a recent infection with yellow fever. It has been known for a long time that monkeys are reservoirs for yellow fever, and the transmission of the disease from monkeys to man depends on the frequency with which the mosquitoes that bite monkeys will also bite man. It thus appears that Uganda is the critical area for any future spread of yellow fever eastwards.

Yellow fever virus and antibodies to yellow fever have been found in other primates, including bush-babies and pottos (Haddow and Ellice, 1964), and in bats (Williams, Simpson, and Shepherd, 1964), and these must all be regarded as a potential source of the disease in man. It has even been suggested that reptiles should not be overlooked as potential reservoirs of yellow fever virus as *Aedes* mosquitoes bite them (McClelland and Weitz, 1963).

Yellow fever can be prevented by inoculation, but this is not always possible in well-dispersed rural populations of people who are suspicious of modern medicine. Much effort has been devoted to eradicating the mosquito vectors by the use of insecticides, but as is usual resistant strains of the mosquito tend to spread through the population. The genetics of these resistant strains is often remarkably simple; in *Aedes aegypti* resistance to DDT is controlled by major genes (Coker, 1966). Another approach to control of *Aedes aegypti* populations is through selection of genotypes that produce an excess of males. Mass breeding of such genotypes and their release in natural populations should not only reduce the population but also reduce the frequency of biting as the males cannot bite (Hickey and Craig, 1966).

In 1959 and later o'nyong nyong fever spread as an epidemic across Uganda into Kenya and Tanzania affecting, it has been estimated, about five million people (Williams *et al.*, 1965). The word 'o'nyong nyong' is Acholi for 'joint breaker' which describes the severe joint pains, often accompanied with a rash, that the fever causes. The arbovirus causing o'nyong nyong is transmitted by *Anopheles* mosquitoes of the same species that transmit malaria, and it would appear that the probability of the disease is higher in areas subject to malaria than elsewhere. The disease resembles the several known forms of dengue, which, however, has not been positively identified in tropical Africa, a suspected epidemic in Tanzania having been shown to be due to a virus related to the one causing o'nyong nyong (Williams and Woodall, 1964). O'nyong nyong is rarely a killing disease but its effects impart a considerable increase in morbidity to populations that are already suffering from malnutrition, malaria, and other diseases. The search for the vector and the nature of the arbovirus causing o'nyong nyong led to the discovery of other viruses which at least at present seem to be of minor epidemiological importance (Woodall and Williams, 1967).

Zika virus, so named because of its first discovery in the Zika Forest of Uganda, is transmitted by *Aedes africanus*, a mosquito that is especially associated with forest. Both man and monkeys can be infected. The virus causes a rash and pains throughout the body (Simpson, 1964). Mosquitoes carrying the virus frequently swarm in the evening above the canopy of the forest and it is under these conditions that it is likely that they would be carried considerable distances by air currents (Haddow, Williams *et al.*, 1964).

As already mentioned, filariasis is now possibly the most widespread mosquito-borne disease in the world in terms of the morbidity and mortality that it causes. The disease is transmitted by the mosquito, *Culex pipiens fatigans*, a species that is especially associated with towns and cities with poor sanitation, and also by various species of *Anopheles*. The pathogens are nematodes, *Wuchereria bancrofti*, which are extremely persistent in the host so that some people are more or less permanently affected. The larvae of *Wuchereria* leave the proboscis of the mosquito when it contacts the warm skin of a man, and then enter through the puncture in the skin made by the mosquito as it feeds. Metamorphosis of the larvae to adults takes place in lymphatic tissue and after breeding the pre-larvae, or microfilariae, concentrate in the lung, migrating to the peripheral blood vessels in the middle of the night. This periodicity is thus associated with the biting cycle of the mosquito vector which bites at night and takes up the microfilariae as it sucks blood. Exactly how the periodicity of movement of the microfilariae and the biting behaviour of the mosquito are synchronized is not known, but possibly changes in the temperature of the blood associated with resting and activity act as a stimulus to the microfilariae. Not all forms of *Wuchereria* are periodic in this way, but the periodic form seems to occur throughout the tropics. The disease has been effectively treated with drugs in The Gambia (McGregor and Gilles, 1960) and elsewhere; the filariasis-carrying mosquitoes have been subjected to programmes of eradication using the usual methods and with the usual conflicting results that seem such a feature of mosquito-control programmes.

Onchocerciasis is caused by an infection with a nematode, *Onchocerca volvulus*, which resembles the one causing filariasis. It is transmitted by flies of the genus *Simulium*, which consists of a complex of similar species, some of which bite man while others do not. The larvae of *Simulium* are aquatic and occur chiefly in streams, the later larval stages and the pupae of certain species being closely associated with freshwater crabs and the nymphs of mayflies. The disease causes eye defects (including blindness) and skin lesions which may lead to further complications. In a forest village in Cameroon it has been found that the potential for transmission of the disease is higher in the 11–30 age group than in other age groups, and that women are less of a source of transmission than men (Duke and Moore, 1968). It appears that in West Africa there are two strains of *Onchocerca volvulus*, each associated with a physiological form of the vector *Simulium damnosum*. One of these strains is associated with the West African rain forest area, and the other with the savanna to the north. It has been suggested that the two strains of the pathogen differ in their effect on the human host and in their susceptibility to treatment by drugs (Duke, Lewis, and Moore, 1966). The vectors of onchocerciasis breed in running water and the changing patterns of the use of running water in tropical Africa may be expected to alter the frequency and distribution of the disease. Evidently the construction of dams has in some cases increased the possible breeding sites of *Simulium* by creating fast-running spillways, while the flooding out of rapids may have decreased the available breeding sites (Raybould, 1968). Many countries in Africa have in recent years received large numbers of political refugees from neighbouring countries, and Wegesa (1968) has shown that refugees from Mozambique arriving in Tanzania make contact with the disease for the first time. Mass movements of people from one area to another are creating situations of considerable importance for those concerned with the prevention of disease.

Trypanosomiasis as a disease of cattle has been discussed in Chapter 7. In man the disease is usually known as sleeping sickness. The pathogens are various species of Protozoa of the genus *Trypanosoma*, some of which do not affect man, or at least very rarely. Part of the life cycle of the trypanosomes takes place in tsetse flies, *Glossina*, and they are transmitted to man and other animals when the fly bites in order to suck blood. The disease is not so important in man as it used to be. At the beginning of the century there were epidemics in the Congo and around the shores of Lake Victoria. In Uganda in particular many people were moved from the danger zones, which included the islands of Lake Victoria, which even today are not as densely populated as they were at one time. Two of the species of pathogen that affect man, *T. rhodesiense* and *T. gambiense*, are distinguishable mainly by the way they survive and reproduce in rats and in their susceptibility to drugs. In Uganda both of these species have undergone fluctuations in abundance since the major epidemics at the beginning of the century, and at present it appears that *T. gambiense* has replaced *T. rhodesiense* (Robertson and Baker, 1958). As mentioned in Chapter 7, large numbers of wild mammals, the reservoir hosts of the disease, have been killed, and extensive areas of bush cleared, in attempts to eradicate the tsetse flies. These efforts have had only limited success and it can be predicted that some species of tsetse flies will become more and more adapted to cultivated areas. Much effort has been devoted to training junior control staff in the methods of tsetse fly eradication, and there is a book designed for use in Northern Nigeria that not only describes how the flies can be identified and destroyed, but also provides drawings showing how wild mammals can be recognized by their tracks and droppings (Davies, 1967).

Schistosomiasis, often called Bilharzia, is one of the most widespread and debilitating diseases in tropical Africa. It is caused by blood flukes, *Schistosoma haematobium* and *S. mansoni*, which enter the body through the skin from contaminated water. The first part of the life cycle of these flukes takes place inside aquatic snails, *S. haematobium* being associated with snails of the genus *Bulinus*, and *S. mansoni* with *Biomphalaria*. Several species in each group of snails are involved and the relative importance of the two forms of the disease varies in different parts of Africa. Many other mammals are also infected with schistosomiasis and it is possible that there is some transmission between other mammals and man, although in general the species of *Schistosoma* differ in different species of mammals. *S. mansoni* affects the blood system of the intestine and

S. haematobium that of the urinary system. The disease is rarely a killer by itself but many people suffering from it also suffer from other diseases, including malnutrition, and its effect is mainly debilitating. In some areas almost all people are infected, but relatively few exhibit severe symptoms. This has led to considerable controversy as to what should be done about the disease, possibly explaining why research on schistosomiasis has tended to lag behind that on other common diseases, such as malaria. Indeed in Africa much of the research on the snail hosts of schistosomiasis is in the descriptive natural history stage. Almost everything published on the disease in recent years indicates that it is holding its own throughout tropical Africa, and in some areas spreading. The main obstacle to the eradication of the disease in even quite small areas is the habits of the people: fresh water is repeatedly contaminated when they urinate and defecate into it, and in doing so the life cycle of the flukes is perpetuated as the eggs are taken back to the water and the snails infected. It has been argued that further research on the disease will achieve little, and that what is needed is a massive programme of persuading people to become sanitary (Newsome, 1959).

The high incidence of infection with *S. haematobium* in children in the 6–12 age group seems partly attributable to indiscriminate urination while in or near water (Jordan, 1961), particularly among small boys who are notoriously careless in this matter, both in Africa and elsewhere. It would appear unlikely that people would habitually urinate in water from which they drink or in which they wash (although one cannot be certain about this), and it is more probable that infected urine is introduced into water under other circumstances.

There is evidence that schistosomiasis has increased and spread in areas where irrigation schemes have been developed, including estates devoted to the cultivation of a single crop and where a large labour force is employed (Sturrock, 1966; Foster, 1967a, 1967b, 1967c). Attempts have been made to estimate the effects of the disease on the working efficiency of the employees and to relate the cost of eradicating the disease to possible increases in production as a result of an improved ability to work. A detailed review of advances in knowledge of schistosomiasis in East Africa ends with

the suggestion that the disease could be controlled by using molluscicides against the host snails, by extending chemotherapy to
children, who are particularly liable to infection, and by the provision of protected water (Webbe and Jordan, 1966). In the discussion
following the review, which was delivered at a meeting of the Royal
Society of Tropical Medicine and Hygiene, C. A. Wright suggested
that the provision of protected water and sanitary facilities should
be in a form that is acceptable to the people. He went on to say
that there is a sociological problem and that it is essential that a
clear idea is obtained as to what constitutes acceptable washing and
latrine facilities, as without this much money and time can be wasted.

The eggs of *Schistosoma haematobium* are passed out in the urine
and there is a diurnal cycle in the number of eggs passed, the peak
being reached in the early afternoon. Blood cells are also passed
with the urine and in severe cases loss of blood may be heavy and
the urine red in colour. Table 20 shows the relationship between the
number of eggs being excreted in the urine and the amount of blood
lost in people in a Sukuma village in Tanzania. Blood loss is directly
proportional to the number of eggs excreted, but except in those few
individuals excreting large numbers of eggs the loss of blood is
unlikely to have been a major cause of anaemia. On the other hand
most of the people in this area that are infected with schistosomiasis
also suffer from other blood parasites: in Sukumaland between a half
and three-quarters, depending on age, are also infected with hookworm, which can cause severe anaemia.

Table 21 shows the incidence of infection with schistosomiasis in
relation to age among people in the same area. The average number
of eggs excreted in the urine is also shown. Only about a quarter of
the very young children were infected, but after the age of five,
between a half and three-quarters of the people were infected.
Judged by the number of eggs being excreted, children between the
age of six and twelve years suffer most severely. It is possible that
the lower infection in adults is related to the development of some
degree of immunity to the parasite, but the high rates of infection
in children are probably partly accounted for by urinating as they
play in water.

Schistosomiasis can be treated with drugs which act as a poison
to the parasites. Until recently many of the drugs used simply

suppressed the disease without actually eradicating it, but it now seems that the disease can be cured by relatively simple means. Morbidity is difficult to assess in a chronic disease like schistosomiasis, but there is evidence that treatment of infected children near Mwanza in Tanzania resulted in an improvement in their position at school (Jordan and Randall, 1962). Antimony therapy (in the form of Astiban) is frequently used as a treatment, and in the course of such treatment of thirty-six Asian schoolboys infected with *S. mansoni* at Mwanza it was found that the effectiveness of the treatment varied significantly with the diet of the boys, as shown in Table 22. Many Asians are vegetarians and the results indicate that these responded less well to treatment than boys that included meat in their diet. These results are difficult to explain although it is known that in mice infected with *S. mansoni* the efficacy of antimony therapy depends on the diet the animals have received.

Attempts to eradicate schistosomiasis by destroying the snail hosts have repeatedly been made, but thus far with limited success. One problem is that *Bulinus* snails can aestivate in dry mud and so even the draining of swamps and ponds fails to eradicate them. Various molluscicides have been used, but these often damage other animals and plants in the water. Strangely enough it appears that pollution of the water with organic wastes can substantially reduce the snail population, and it has been suggested that sisal waste which is apparently toxic to snails, and which in Tanzania is often dumped into rivers and streams, might be used as a molluscicide (Otieno, 1966). Thus unlike the situation in Europe and North America, in Africa pollution of the water can possibly improve the health of the population by destroying snails and other animals that are intermediate hosts or vectors of human disease.

Research has also been initiated on the genetics of the snails and there is evidence that some of the genotypes within a population have different susceptibility to infection by schistosomes. It is thought that by breeding certain strains of snails it might be possible to introduce the more resistant genotypes into natural populations so that they displace the existing snails. But the idea depends upon the unlikely assumption that the schistosomes themselves will not become adapted to the new strains.

Many people in tropical Africa are anaemic as the result of the presence of several different blood parasites and of a deficiency of protein in the diet. In Gambian villages anaemia is especially associated with heavy hookworm infections in men, but not in women (Topley, 1968a, 1968b). Results of tests for schistosomiasis in samples of people from many parts of Africa have also indicated that hookworm infections are important in anaemia, and one report (Jordan and Randall, 1962) describes a significant association between hookworm infection and schistosomiasis caused by *S. mansoni*. Hookworm larvae are picked up when a person walks barefoot on infected ground, while schistosomiasis is acquired from infected water. Thus the sources of the two diseases are different and this perhaps suggests that an individual with one disease is so weakened that he is more likely to acquire and suffer significantly from the other. This kind of pattern of infection is probably of common occurrence.

There are many other diseases in tropical Africa, including most of those found elsewhere in the world, and from birth to death the average person suffers chronically and lives in constant fear of being infected with a killing or crippling disease. Epidemics of smallpox, measles, and a host of conditions caused by arboviruses are likely to break out at any time, and may result in high mortality rates before the attention of the medical authorities is called and some attempt is made to arrest the spread of the disease. Chronic diseases, such as leprosy, tend to occur more in some areas than in others, and there is a wide spectrum of minor illnesses which add to the hazards of everyday life. One of the most common of the minor diseases is trachoma, a virus infection of the eye which can cause blindness, and which is believed by some to be the commonest disease in the world (Werner *et al.*, 1964). Blister beetles of various species can become extremely abundant in the wet season. When squashed on the skin they cause a form of dermatitis (Giglioli, 1965), and may give rise to blisters around the eye which are most uncomfortable. There are fly larvae which by a variety of methods find their way to the skin and bore into the flesh causing ugly and painful sores, thus providing sites for additional infections.

It is sometimes said that cancer, heart diseases, and tuberculosis are less frequent in Africa than in temperate regions, but it is more probable that they have been overlooked, as have many of the inherited diseases, simply because there are so many other more obvious conditions that demand the attention. Thus in 1953 virtually nothing was known about the frequency of tuberculosis in Ghana, but after a unit had been set up to survey the situation in the country it was found that there was an overall morbidity rate of 1·3 per cent and that the disease is more prevalent in the rural coastal area than in towns where, on the basis of findings elsewhere, it might be expected to be more frequent (Koch and Laing, 1962).

The future pattern of disease transmission in tropical Africa is a matter for speculation, but it would seem likely that with rising human numbers the towns and cities are likely to become the major centres of outbreaks. Domestic dogs are becoming a major public health problem in African towns. They are poorly fed and outbreaks of disease among them are frequent. Dogs can transmit a variety of diseases, including rabies. Rabies is probably a much more common cause of death in people than is generally supposed.

Published reviews of diseases in tropical Africa repeatedly reach the conclusion that the major problem is persuading people to be sanitary. Those concerned with public health are constantly frustrated by the widespread tendency among the people to urinate and defecate in public places and at will, rather than at well-defined private places. It remains, however, a matter for speculation whether the single act of providing lavatories for everyone will have a significant effect on the present pattern of disease transmission.

CHAPTER 10

Natural Selection and Genetics

The individuals that make up a population of organisms differ from each other in a wide variety of features, morphological, physiological, and behavioural. Many of these differences are determined by the direct effects of the environment on the individual, but others are inherited from the parents. Man is no exception and the human population is immensely variable, many of the variations being hereditary. Some obvious features in people, such as size and proportions, are determined by the combined effects of the environment and genes. Other features, such as skin colour and blood group, are genetic and are not affected directly by the environment. But the distribution and frequency with which genetic features occur is in most cases determined by the environment in which the population is living.

The genetically determined variation in man arises to a large extent from pressures exerted by the environment through the process of natural selection. It is also determined by complex mating systems which result in non-random breeding, and by movements of individuals and populations from one area to another over relatively short periods of time. Natural selection is the non-random and therefore selective elimination of genes from the population. The elimination of a gene involves the death of the individual possessing it. In genetic terms the age of death is of great importance. When children die they have not transmitted their genes to the next generation, but the death of an adult, especially of an old person, may occur after reproduction, and hence after genes have been transmitted to the next generation. The capacity of an individual to transmit genes to the next generation is called the fitness of the individual. This term must not be confused with physical fitness: many individuals in poor health leave a lot of children and thus have a high fitness. An Olympic athlete who does not marry and produce children has a fitness of zero, but a Gambian peasant, suffering from malaria, hookworm, and malnutrition, with ten children, and two pregnant wives has a high genetic fitness value.

The present diversity of human populations is largely the result of natural selection acting in response to the environment. This explains why there is so much geographical variation in the appearance of people in different parts of the world. If the environment changes there may be a change in gene frequency in the population, and such a change is what is known as evolution. Man is constantly subjected to natural selection and hence to the possibility of evolution. The introduction of carbohydrate staple foods into Africa from elsewhere and the widespread eradication of malaria as a killing disease are examples of environmental changes that have undoubtedly affected the genetic structure of the population of Africa, although it must be admitted that it would be difficult to measure in precise terms exactly what has happened. The human population of tropical Africa is increasing very rapidly, but the rate of increase is not as high as the potential for increase. As shown in earlier chapters, many children die before the age of reproduction, and it can be assumed that much of this mortality is selective. Those that survive transmit their genes to the next generation and the process is repeated generation after generation, changes in the probability of death occurring whenever the possible causes of death change.

In tropical Africa, and elsewhere in the world, there appear to be two features of the environment that affect the selective mortality among individuals in human populations. These are the efficiency with which the available food resources are utilized and the response to disease. It is possible that at one time predatory animals resulted in considerable selective mortality, but this hazard is nowadays negligible, deaths from motor car accidents being far more frequent than deaths from snake bites. Indeed it would seem that disease is by far the most important feature of the environment that affects the genetic diversity of man. If so, it follows that the varied programmes designed to eliminate disease must exert a considerable effect on the genetic structure of human populations. The use of drugs, vaccines, inoculations, and all the preventive measures that are now known, must result in a change in the individual's probability of death, and hence a change in the genetic structure of the population. In general terms the war against disease should result in an increase in the genetic variance as many people now survive who under former ecological circumstances would have died before reproducing.

Genetic variation in man may be continuous or discontinuous. The distribution of human birth weights is an example of continuous variation. In a large sample the frequency of birth weights approximates a normal distribution. Very heavy and very light babies die at or shortly after birth, and it is evident that the optimal weight is at the mode of the distribution. Birth weight is partly genetically and partly environmentally determined and there is constant selection against abnormally heavy and light babies. Other examples of continuous variation are adult height and skin colour. Indeed most genetically determined human traits have a continuous distribution. Such traits are determined by the combined effects of several genes at different loci, and the inheritance of the traits is thus polygenic. From the standpoint of genetic analysis polygenic traits are difficult to deal with, but it is possible to show that the tendencies are transmitted from generation to generation, and that there are geographical components to their occurrence: both human height and skin colour vary markedly in different parts of the world.

The timing of tooth eruption varies among people in different parts of the world. Permanent tooth eruption occurs earlier in Africans than in Europeans (Roberts, 1969), but the eruption of deciduous teeth occurs more slowly in African than in European children, as shown in Table 23. African children lag behind European children in the number of erupted teeth for the first eighteen months, but thereafter they catch up and by the age of two years there is little difference between them. This suggests that the rate of development of deciduous teeth among different groups of people is genetically determined.

Discontinuous variation in which there are two or more distinct phenotypes in the population is rather less common than continuous variation, but it is much more amenable to genetic analysis and is less subject to direct environmental influence. The eyes of Europeans may be brown, grey, or blue; other colours occur but the variation is essentially discontinuous. Africans have dark brown eyes which vary in shade between individuals; other contrasting colours are extremely rare, but they do occur for Erasmus Harland informs me that he has seen two Nilotic Ugandans, a brother and a sister, with blue eyes. Most of the known discontinuous variation in man is not obvious as it involves blood groups, abnormal haemoglobins, and differences in seeing, tasting, and smelling abilities.

The existence of discontinuous variation within a population is usually referred to as polymorphism, which is defined as the occurrence in the same population of two or more distinct genetically determined phenotypes in such proportions that the rarest of them cannot be maintained by recurrent mutation alone. The last part of the definition is important as it excludes numerous rare mutants, although it is not always possible to say whether a rare phenotype is maintained by recurrent mutation or by natural selection. Thus it would seem that the occurrence of haemophilia in human populations is mainly through recurrent mutation, but the situation is complex as the gene is sex-linked, and usually expresses itself only in males. Females can be carriers of the gene but need show no evidence of the disease which will, however, appear in some of their male offspring. Albinism in man is determined independently by several different genes and thus it is not possible to decide whether, for instance, albino Africans constitute an example of polymorphism or whether they occur as recurrent mutations. A polymorphic trait can be maintained in the population if the fitness of the heterozygotes is greater than that of either of the homozygotes or if the fitness of a phenotype varies with its frequency in the population. There is much evidence from other animals that the second possibility is of widespread occurrence, the most striking examples being in polymorphic mimetic butterflies, in which the polymorphism is maintained by selective predation. Numerous examples of polymorphism have been discovered in man, many of them involving alternative forms of haemoglobin and different blood groups, the ABO system being the best known.

In man disease can operate as a selective factor, but only if the selective mortality takes place before the completion of reproduction. Some diseases do not normally develop until the individual is past the age of reproduction. These cannot act selectively, but it is possible that the age at which individuals become susceptible to disease has been constantly pushed back by the application of modern medicine. Indeed an important achievement of modern medicine has been to postpone the onset of many diseases until later in life such that nowadays many individuals die only after they have reproduced. It would seem that most infant mortality is selective in terms of relative ability to resist the effects of various diseases.

Almost all the numerous genes that have been identified in man vary in frequency from place to place, sometimes even over quite short distances. Such variations have been repeatedly reported for other animals and plants and they reflect responses to different selection pressures imposed by the environment. If groups of organisms are more or less isolated from one another by ecological and geographical barriers the variation in gene frequency from place to place is even more striking. In man there is an additional factor that promotes isolation: the tendency of ethnic groups to breed among themselves and not with other ethnic groups. This mode of breeding is perhaps better developed in Africa than anywhere else in the world.

Many diseases are transmitted more rapidly and thus affect a higher proportion of the population in crowded areas than in areas where the people are well dispersed. Variations in population density should, therefore, be an additional factor affecting the frequency of genes that are associated with disease.

One approach to estimating local variations in selection in response to disease is to try and detect local variations in morbidity, mortality, and immunity. Roberts (1965) gives an example of this for immunity to tuberculosis in Northern Nigeria. It is not known for certain that there are genetic factors associated with the probability of dying from tuberculosis, but if there are the disease would act as a selective agent. Roberts found a cline or gradient of diminishing frequency of immunity outwards from an urban area to rural areas, which suggests differential contact with tuberculosis, greatest in the more densely populated urban area and least in the remote rural villages. Tuberculosis is usually associated with people living in crowded conditions and the cline in immunity shows that more people had been exposed to the disease in the town than in the villages.

In another survey in the same part of Nigeria, Roberts (1965) cites the work of P. Collard on local variations in the frequency of infection with *Schistosoma haematobium* in villages scattered over an area of about 1800 km². The frequency of infection varied markedly from village to village, but there was no cline or gradient, and the probability of infection was presumably associated with the quality of the local water supply. The population in this area is thus not homogeneous in its probability of exposure to the disease and this might impart differences in natural selection if the disease is responsible for even a small amount of mortality.

Numerous other examples of this sort have been documented and it would seem likely that local variations in intensity of a disease would affect the frequency of genes that impart some degree of resistance. Genetic resistance is maintained most effectively in a sedentary population that is repeatedly exposed to disease. Newly introduced diseases are often catastrophic as the population has not evolved the appropriate resistance.

There was a time when anthropologists favoured the use of variations in the frequency of blood group and abnormal haemo-globin genes as a means of tracing the ethnic origin of people in different areas, and in particular as a means of defining genetic differences in the races of man. It was assumed that these genetic traits were conservative or neutral in effect and thus provided evidence as to where people had come from, as the traits were unlikely to have undergone changes in response to natural selection. This view is still held by a minority of anthropologists. Geneticists have appreciated that the existence of distinct phenotypes in a population, together with local or geographical variations in the frequency of phenotypes, can be explained in terms of natural selection, and have repeatedly urged that the different phenotypes are likely to be correlated with the occurrence and intensity of diseases (Ford, 1965). Since the discovery by Allison (1954a, 1954b, 1954c) that the distribution and frequency of the sickle cell trait, one of the abnormal haemoglobins, is correlated with the occurrence and intensity of malaria caused by *Plasmodium falciparum*, evidence has accumulated that other abnormal haemoglobins and some of the blood groups are also associated with the presence of certain diseases.

The foetal haemoglobin in man (haemoglobin F) is replaced by the normal type A soon after birth, but in some people another type, S, partly or almost completely replaces A. There are thus three types of individual: normal homozygotes with the genotype Hb^AHb^A, homozygotes with the genotype Hb^SHb^S, and heterozygotes Hb^AHb^S. Individuals that are homozygous Hb^SHb^S have a poor expectation of life, four out of five dying of anaemia in childhood and the remainder rarely surviving to reproduce, and hence this genotype has a fitness that is very close to zero. In the absence of normal haemoglobin the red blood cells of such individuals become sickle-shaped and tend to block the capillaries and in consequence are phagocytosed and cause anaemia (Ford, 1965). Heterozygous Hb^AHb^S people produce sickle-shaped blood cells only under abnormal conditions in which the oxygen pressure is reduced, and to all intents and purposes they are quite normal. The red blood cells of such people assume the sickle shape if a drop of blood is placed under reduced oxygen tension. The strong selection against the homozygous sicklers immediately suggests that either the mutation rate is extremely high or that the heterozygotes have some advantage over the homozygous non-sicklers. Heterozygote frequencies of up to 40 per cent occur in some parts of Africa, and in many areas the frequency is around 20 per cent, and it follows from this alone that the explanation of the sickle cell trait must be sought in terms of heterozygote advantage. The distribution of the sickle cell gene (Fig. 9) includes the whole of tropical Africa, Madagascar, parts of Arabia, the Middle East, and southern Europe (Livingstone, 1965). It is most frequent in negroids, but it is not a racial feature as it also occurs in caucasoids (south Europeans and Arabs).

The demonstration by Allison that the distribution and frequency of Hb^AHb^S individuals is associated with that of malaria caused by *Plasmodium falciparum* has been repeatedly confirmed, and there is also some experimental evidence that these heterozygotes are more resistant to malarial infections than Hb^AHb^A homozygotes. It has been shown that children who die from heavy malarial infection are nearly always non-sicklers. Marked regional variations in the frequency of the heterozygotes are correlated with the intensity of malaria and with human population densities, which of course also affect the probability of transmission of the disease, and also with the development of agriculture which often results in an increase in the intensity of malaria by providing suitable breeding places for the vectors (Wiesenfeld, 1967; Livingstone, 1958a, 1958b, 1960, 1961,

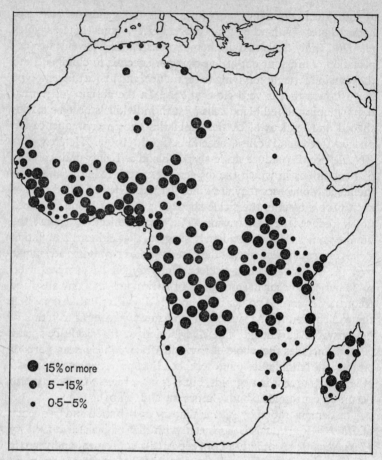

15% or more
5–15%
0·5–5%

Fig. 9 Percentage incidence of individuals with haemoglobin S in populations in Africa. (*From Livingstone, 1965.*)

1962). The present frequency of the heterozygotes in different parts of Africa is thus to be interpreted in terms of relatively recent ecological changes in the area associated with the spread of agriculture, rising human population densities, and, in many areas, the suppression of malaria through the use of drugs. Repeated sampling of the human population should produce evidence of changes in the frequency of the heterozygotes in response to changes in their

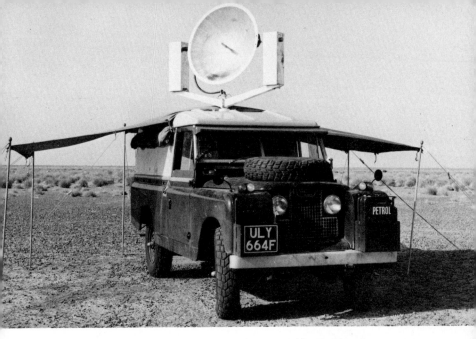

13 Radar equipment mounted on a Land-Rover used in tracking the movements of locusts. Niger, October 1968.

Larvae of the moth, *Spodoptera exempta,* feeding on finger millet. These larvae are often called army-worms because they frequently occur in vast numbers and move from place to place consuming the leaves and stems of grain crops and grasses and causing an immense amount of damage. The fully-grown larva is about 23 mm long.

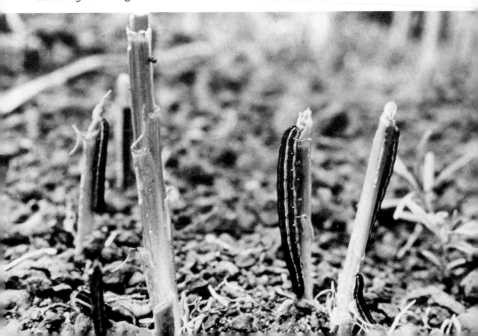

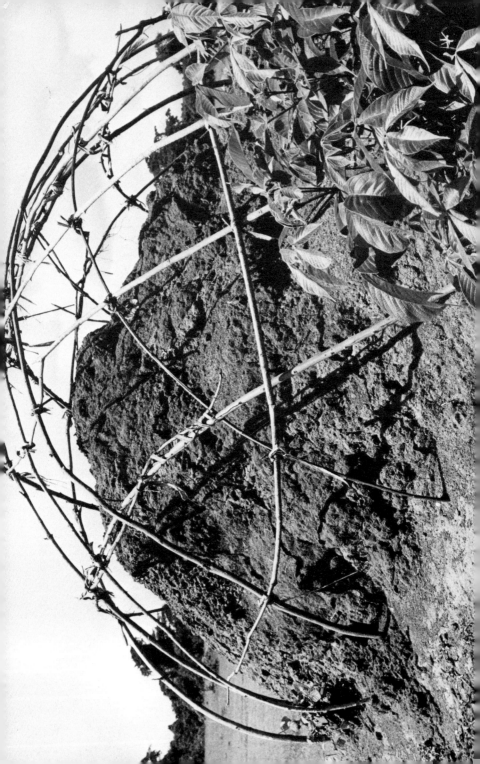

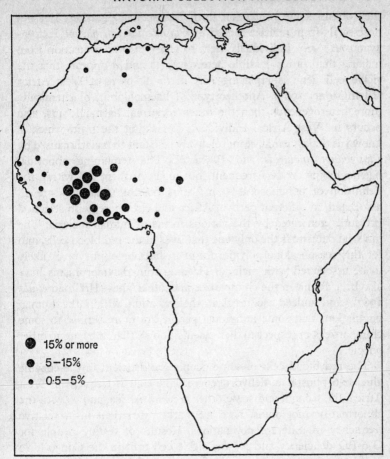

15% or more
5–15%
0·5–5%

Fig. 10 Percentage incidence of individuals with haemoglobin C in populations in Africa. (*From Livingstone, 1965.*)

selective values associated with either increases or decreases in the intensity of malaria as a killing disease.

In West Africa there is another abnormal haemoglobin (haemoglobin C) which is allelic to Hb^A and Hb^S. The distribution and frequency of haemoglobin C is shown in Fig. 10. Individuals with the genotypes $Hb^C Hb^C$ and $Hb^S Hb^C$ suffer from anaemia and it appears that $Hb^A Hb^C$ heterozygotes are at a selective advantage as

14 A trap built over a termite mound. After heavy rain winged termites emerge from the mound and are collected from banana leaves placed over the frame. Termites are highly esteemed as food and many mounds are individually owned.

they obtain some protection from *Plasmodium* parasites, but not necessarily from malaria caused by *Plasmodium falciparum*. Heterozygous *Hb^AHb^S* individuals seem to enjoy greater protection from malaria than other possible heterozygotes and it appears that the sickle cell gene is replacing *Hb^C* in many parts of West Africa (Livingstone, 1965). Another type of haemoglobin, biochemically more heterogeneous than the other abnormal haemoglobins, also occurs in West Africa. Individuals possessing the trait, which is known as thalassaemia, seem relatively resistant to malaria caused by *Plasmodium malariae* and *P. vivax*. The remaining abnormal haemoglobins are less frequent, but many of them fall within the definition of polymorphism, and it is possible that they are all associated, in different parts of Africa and elsewhere, with selection pressures generated by the various forms of human malaria. The malarial parasite is the only one that lives in the red blood cells, and for this reason alone polymorphism in haemoglobin type is likely to be associated with malaria. Haemoglobin polymorphisms have also been found in the chimpanzee and other apes (Hoffman *et al.*, 1967), and indeed, so great is the variation within the human population, that some individual people are more similar to some chimpanzees in respect to their haemoglobins than they are to other people.

The red blood cells of some people are deficient in the enzyme glucose-6-phosphate dehydrogenase. The trait is frequent in West Africa, the Congo, and some other areas of Africa, and as with the abnormal haemoglobins there are marked variations in its relative frequency in different populations. Results of testing people for G-6-PD deficiency and for the sickle cell trait in the Congo have confirmed that variations in the frequency of the two traits are correlated (Motulsky *et al.*, 1966). Examination of pedigrees in the Gambian village of Keneba has confirmed that the trait is sex-linked and is on the X chromosome (Knox and McGregor, 1965). There is selection against the gene since some heterozygotes and homozygotes develop haemolytic disease of the newborn, while in later life other conditions, not at present fully understood, but associated with certain items of diet, may develop (Allison, 1969). However the trait is too frequent to be maintained by recurrent mutation and there is increasing evidence that individuals possessing it are to some extent protected against malaria caused by *Plasmodium falciparum*. The evidence thus far obtained is simply that variations in the frequency of G-6-PD deficient individuals are correlated with variations in the frequency of heterozygous sicklers who are known to be more resistant to malaria. This sex-linked trait is undoubtedly an example of polymorphism, but the mode of balance (if indeed it is balanced) has not yet been established.

Most mammals are effectively colour blind, but man and the apes are unusual in that they can perceive colour. But not all humans have full colour vision. Throughout the world red-green colour blindness occurs at a variable relative frequency in the population. The trait is sex-linked and since it rarely exceeds 10 per cent in males its frequency in females is very low. There seem to be several alleles associated with colour blindness which together give the red-green deficiency, and it has been customary to group them to obtain an overall estimate of the frequency of the phenotype. Red-green colour blindness reaches its highest frequency in Europeans. In southern England about 8 per cent of all males and slightly more than the expected 0·64 per cent of all females are colour blind (Ford, 1965). The slight excess of females over the expected with the trait is possibly accounted for by there being some heterozygous colour-blind females.

The usual way of testing for colour blindness is to ask people the numbers on the plates published by Ishihara (1964). People with red-green colour blindness either cannot read some of the numbers or read different numbers from people with normal vision. The incorporation of plates which involve the tracing of a winding line has enabled the testing of people who are unable to read numbers. The subject is simply asked to trace the winding line or the 'snake' across the page, a task which is attempted with interest in Africa as most people are familiar with snakes. The results of attempts to trace the line are comparable to those obtained in attempts to read the numbers. The Ishihara tests have been extensively used in Africa and normally give satisfactory results.

Roberts (1967) has summarized the results of testing for red-green colour blindness among Africans. As shown in Table 24 the trait occurs in about two per cent of the males in almost all places in Africa where tests have been conducted. This is a much lower frequency than among Europeans, but the most striking feature is the lack of geographical variation in the frequency of the trait. This is in marked contrast to other polymorphisms and is difficult to explain. The trait is of course far too frequent to be caused by recurrent mutation. Even among the people that live in conspicuously different environments, such as forest and savanna, red-green colour blindness occurs at about the same frequency. As already mentioned, the genetic control of the trait is somewhat complicated, but it appears that two series of multiple alleles are involved, one responsible for red and the other for green visual deficiencies. These two series occur at different loci and are rather closely linked to the locus that determines G-6-PD deficiency, but there is not of course any suggestion that similar ecological conditions are associated with the two traits.

The most likely adaptive significance of red-green colour blindness is to be sought in terms of frequency-dependent selection. Such selection favours the maintenance of certain phenotypes in the population providing their frequency does not exceed a certain value. Put differently the phenotypes are at a selective advantage provided they remain relatively rare. Ford (1965) suggests that individuals that are red-green colour blind are able to perceive certain features of the environment that people with normal vision have difficulty over. He mentions in particular the ability of colour-blind people to find cryptic natural objects more efficiently than people with normal vision. Unfortunately there seems to be no experimental evidence in support of this hypothesis, but it is theoretically possible that such a polymorphism could be advantageous in certain environments, although it does not explain the stability of the frequency over vast areas of Africa. It has also been suggested that the trait has increased in frequency among modern man because there is no longer selection against it (Post, 1962), but as pointed out by Ford (1965), this view must be wrong as the trait could not have reached its present status unless there were some selective advantage to it. But the postulated selective advantage remains obscure.

About thirteen different blood groups are known in man, and there are a number of others whose frequency is so low that they probably represent recurrent mutations. All the common blood groups vary in relative frequency in different areas of the world. The existence and importance of blood groups in operations involving blood transfusions has been known for a long time, and it is also known that they are genetically determined by clusters of multiple alleles. They were for long regarded as being of neutral selective value and were thus frequently used as a means of defining groups and races of people. E. B. Ford has repeatedly argued that they constitute an example of balanced polymorphism and that their existence and relative frequency in the population must be determined by natural selection, probably in the form of responses to specific human diseases. Similar blood groups occur in monkeys and apes.

The best known blood groups are the ABO series. These constitute an allelic series which gives four possible phenotypes, O, A, B, or AB, the alleles A and O, and A and A, giving A phenotypes, and the alleles B and O, and B and B, giving B phenotypes. The phenotype of an individual can be tested by using human sera containing anti-A and anti-B proteins. Red cells containing the A antigen agglutinate when exposed to serum containing anti-A, and a similar response occurs when cells containing the B antigen are exposed to anti-B serum. It is thus possible to test quickly large numbers of people. This has been done throughout the world, partly because knowledge of an individual's blood group is important should the need for a blood transfusion arise, and partly because of the interest in regional and ethnic differences in the frequency of the blood groups. It has become increasingly apparent that individuals of different blood groups have a different probability of contracting certain diseases, including broncho-pneumonia, and cancer of the stomach. Some of these diseases are mainly associated with old age after the individual has passed the age of reproduction, and thus this cannot be an important selective factor determining the frequency of the blood groups. It is possible however that the age at which cancer and other diseases associated with old age occur has been pushed back and that at one time the diseases were more prevalent among younger people.

The frequency of the ABO and other blood groups varies throughout Africa, but not as locally and as conspicuously as that of the abnormal haemoglobins. Some of the blood groups are effectively confined to negroids and their presence in pygmies and bushmen is probably the result of recent interbreeding. There is a general feeling that the occurrence and frequency of some of the blood groups might provide indications of the ethnic origin of the negroids, but in view of the strong theoretical reasons for supposing that the blood groups are associated with various diseases, there are difficulties in this approach. It has also been claimed that the present distribution of blood groups can be explained in terms of selection imparted by past epidemics of smallpox and plague, but the subject is highly controversial because although some workers have apparently found a relationship between these diseases and the blood groups others have been unable to confirm it (Allison, 1969).

As is well known there is much geographical variation in the colour of the human skin. The colour of an individual's skin is determined by the amount and distribution of melanin in the epidermis. Negroid skin contains more melanin than caucasoid skin and it is more evenly distributed. Skin colour is genetically determined by a rather complex polygenic system. There is no evidence of polymorphism, provided the occasional occurrence of albinos is excluded. Skin colour is one of the easiest of human traits to recognize and it is notable that variations in skin colour have given rise to the phenomenon of racial discrimination. There is of course a clear tendency for people of similar skin colour to associate and breed together, and this has consequences that affect the genetic structure of the population. Man differs from other animals in that geographically separated populations now repeatedly come face to face with each other. In other animals geographical forms of a species do not meet under circumstances that normally lead to interbreeding or to the possibility of interbreeding.

It has been widely accepted that the melanin pigment in the skin is a protection against exposure to sunlight, thus accounting for the tendency for people to be darker in colour in areas where there is more sunlight, but the evidence for this is by no means conclusive (Blum, 1961). It would appear that a dark skin would be disadvantageous in high temperatures such as those experienced in the savanna and desert areas of Africa, as a dark colour increases the rate of heat gain. A dark skin is less liable to sunburn and to skin cancer than a pale skin, but neither of these conditions is likely to have a conspicuous effect on fitness as they result in death only on extremely rare occasions. Sunlight also initiates a photochemical reaction that results in the synthesis of vitamin D required for the proper development of bone, and a deficiency of this vitamin can result in rickets. The importance of sunlight in maintaining the level of vitamin D in the body is probably not very great as most of the required amount appears to be obtained from the diet. But in areas where the diet is poor in vitamin D exposure to sunlight could be advantageous. It is however difficult to relate the colour of the skin to the probability of death from rickets. The disease is especially prevalent among growing children and there is a possibility that a darker skin may be advantageous. It has also been suggested that the skin colour is cryptic and that people living in forested areas tend to be darker than those living in more open places.

Thus although there are strong theoretical reasons for supposing that skin colour is adaptive, the significance of the remarkable geographical variation in colour that occurs in man remains elusive. It is odd that pale-skinned people spend much time sitting in the sun in order to become darker, while dark-skinned people will buy preparations which they apply to the skin to make it seem paler.

It has been said that when peoples meet they sometimes fight but they always breed. The repeated movements of people from one part of the world to another in the past 10 000 or so years, and especially in the last few hundred years, have resulted in extensive interbreeding that has affected the genetic structure of populations as we now see them. In Africa the spread of the negroids and their increase in numbers after they became cultivators has resulted not only in the virtual extermination of the pygmies and the bushmen, but also in interbreeding between previously isolated groups. In the last few hundred years Africa has also received relatively large numbers of people from other parts of the world, chiefly the European colonizers and traders from Asia, especially from India, the Middle East, and Arabia. With the marked exception of the Portuguese, who have interbred with the negroids, and possibly also the Arabs who have contributed substantially to the evolution of the Swahili-speaking people of the coastal East Africa, the impact of the Europeans and Asians on the genetic structure of the negroids has been small, far smaller than that of the Spaniards and Portuguese on the indigenous population of South America.

In tropical Africa there is a conspicuous tendency for breeding to occur within the ethnic group. This is sometimes condemned by modern politicians as an undesirable aspect of tribalism, but it is favoured by the community as a whole and even by some politicians. Roberts (1965) has given figures that indicate the amount of inter-mixture of people of different ethnic groups by recording the extent of intermarriage in Nilotic populations consisting of distinct ethnic groups or tribes. In 288 marriages in Dinka villages eight spouses were Nuer and five were Shilluk; in 255 marriages in Shilluk villages five spouses were Dinka and one Nuer. This marriage, or mating, rate can be used to estimate gene flow rates, as shown in Table 25. Almost all the matings were between people of like ethnic groups, and it is tempting to assume that gene flow between the three populations is small. Roberts then goes on to calculate the cumulative effect of these rates over twenty generations, making the assumption that the rates of intermarriage remain constant. His results are reproduced in Table 26 where it can be seen that even with such a low rate of intermixture in each generation each population is rapidly diluted so that, taking the Dinka as an example, only two-thirds of the genes are derived from the original population. Thus even a small ripple on a gene pool can become a wave after a rela-tively small number of breeding generations have elapsed. In this instance it is assumed that natural selection is not operating against the donor ethnic group in its new environment. Thus although in Africa there is a strong tendency to breed within the group, even a small amount of outbreeding can over several generations have conspicuous genetic consequences.

Distance is also an important barrier to interbreeding. Among all peoples there is a marked tendency for breeding to occur with those near by, and such people are of course likely to be more similar genetically than those from distant places. There are numerous other factors that affect the probability of breeding, among them religious beliefs and taboos that are rarely violated by illiterate people, but which are increasingly ignored by people who regard themselves as sophisticated. Assortative mating, or the breeding together of like phenotypes, has been reported in a number of species of animals, including man. The psychological factors involved in assortative mating are not easy to identify, but there is a tendency for men to marry women who have certain features, morphological, intellectual, or economic, that resemble their own. It is possibly more pronounced among Europeans than other peoples in the world. It has been suggested that men like to marry women that look like their own mothers, and there is some evidence for this. This suggests a form of imprinting similar to that which occurs in mate selection among birds. An individual's choice of a mate obviously depends on a variety of factors, not the least of which are availability and willingness. Assortative mating has the effect of increasing the genetic variance of the population by promoting homozygosity. In extreme examples, such as brother–sister matings, deleterious effects may express themselves in the recessive phenotypes of the offspring, and this is probably why matings between close relatives are discouraged by taboos in Africa and elsewhere in the world.

In man and other animals natural selection usually affects the fitness of the individual and not that of the group. Wynne-Edwards (1963) has however interpreted the existence of social and territorial behaviour among 'higher' animals as an adaptation in which competition for space and social status is substituted for direct competition for resources such as food. This behaviour, he says, provides a means by which populations can be self-limiting and in which selection favours the society or group rather than the individual. Developing his theory, Wynne-Edwards cites Carr-Saunders (1922) who suggests that primitive hunters and agriculturalists placed restrictions on their fertility by practising abortion and infanticide, and by abstaining from intercourse, especially during lactation.[1] This, it is argued, limits the size of the group to what is compatible with the available resources. Infanticide was (and possibly still is) practised by African bushmen, young children being left to die in the desert rather than being deliberately killed, and, according to Wynne-Edwards, this adjusted the population to an optimum size.

Wynne-Edwards then goes on to say that the beginnings of the

---

[1] The widespread occurrence of homosexuality in man (and some other animals) might also be a population-regulating mechanism.

agricultural revolution resulted in a displacement of this traditional mode of population regulation and as time passed and the human population expanded the social conventions were abandoned and 'nothing' was acquired in their place. Man began to interact directly with the environment and eventually the conventional means of population control were lost.

The difficulty with this theory is that it does not explain by what manner of process the supposed population-regulating adaptations were lost. If, as suggested by Wynne-Edwards, selection for the group was effective, how can we account for its apparent disappearance in modern man? It now appears that the fertility and the rate of population increase in man are directly correlated with the available resources. Evidence for this is given in Chapter 2 in which it is seen that the high birth and death rates in West African villages are not associated with deliberate social conventions to limit population growth. The habit of abstaining from intercourse while a baby is still feeding at the breast can be explained in terms of individual rather than group selection, as the conception of another child before the first is weaned could result in the death of both, and in some cases the death of the mother as well. Infanticide initially appears to provide evidence for group selection but it could equally be an adaptation associated with the survival of the individual. Thus at times of food shortage there may not be enough food to feed all the adults and the children. If adults were sacrificed the children would die anyway, and hence the death of children can result in the survival of the parents who can of course breed again when ecological conditions become more favourable. It is of interest in this regard that the bushmen (and other peoples practising infanticide) do not usually deliberately kill the children but abandon them so that they starve, and then attribute their death to the will of supernatural powers.

But despite the above considerations it would appear that a form of group selection is in its incipient stages in some parts of the modern world, although not to any significant extent in Africa. Limiting the size of the family by artificial methods of birth control means that a family will not only be able to share the available resources more favourably, but will also be able to substitute other things (some of them not unconnected with status) for a large number of children. Contraception is now being advocated as a social as well as a family necessity and if the habit spreads it will lead to intergroup selection of the kind postulated by Wynne-Edwards, who, however, does not discuss birth control in modern man.

CHAPTER 11

The Ecology of Development

The world has been described as a space ship in which there are fixed amounts of non-renewable (capital) resources, and renewable resources, essentially plants and the organisms that feed on plants. By the process of photosynthesis, green plants convert radiant energy from the sun into chemical energy, which is stored and utilized (directly or indirectly) as food for all other organisms, including man. Almost all organic material produced is utilized and there is little long-term accumulation. Until the relatively recent advent of industrial man the non-renewable resources of the world (coal, oil, minerals, etc.) had not been appreciably utilized as a source of energy, but there is now an unprecedented scramble to use energy from non-renewable resources.

Man's ability to cultivate crops and to domesticate animals, as well as his ability to utilize the stored energy of oil and minerals, sets him apart from other organisms. These unique ecological properties, together with man's ability to control and eradicate diseases, have produced a human population far bigger than that of any other organism of remotely comparable size. It is uncertain when the species we now call *Homo sapiens* first became differentiated, but what is certain is that it took hundreds of thousands of years for the human population to reach its first 1000 million. This was achieved in about 1830, then, in the next hundred years, the population reached 2000 million, and in the next thirty years (in 1960) it reached 3000 million. By 1975 (fifteen years after 1960) the world population should pass the 4000 million mark, and by the turn of the century at least 1000 million people will be added every five years if the present rate of increase is maintained. These figures are of course horrifying and it is obvious that within the next fifty or a hundred years the rate of increase will have to fall, but exactly how this will happen is a matter of speculation. It seems virtually certain that many of us alive today will hear of or experience widespread famine within our lifetime.

Two-thirds of the present population of the world are living in poverty while the remaining third, in the developed nations, are living in comparative luxury. The average person in a developed country uses up non-renewable resources at a rate of between thirty and fifty times that of a person in an under-developed country. For some resources the average rate of utilization is hundreds of times greater than what occurs in an under-developed country: on average an Englishman uses as much steel in a month as a Gambian uses in his lifetime. Hence despite the high rates of increase of the population in under-developed countries the population in developed countries, with a much lower rate of increase, has a much greater impact on the world's resources: the ecological impact of a birth in a developed country is potentially fifty times greater than one in an under-developed country.

All the countries of tropical Africa are officially designated as under-developed and all are striving, in most cases unsuccessfully, to become developed. Put differently, this means that the aim of under-developed countries is to use resources at a rate that is equivalent to that in a developed country. All the countries of tropical Africa produce raw materials, renewable and non-renewable, that are sold to and consumed in developed countries. Just how long this state of affairs can be sustained is anyone's guess. How long, for instance, can Sierra Leone rely upon the export of uncut diamonds and Zambia upon the export of copper ore? Both of these exports depend upon demands for them by developed countries, both resources are non-renewable, and there will come a time when diamonds and copper can no longer be produced in sufficient quantity to interest the business community of the developed countries. When this occurs the present unstable economies of Sierra Leone and Zambia will become even more unstable.

Consider, as a more specific example, the fate of iron ore mined in Africa and exported raw to Britain. The iron is converted into steel and is then used for a variety of industrial purposes, among them the manufacture of motor cars, an industry which keeps thousands of people in Britain in employment and which contributes substantially to the country's economy. The motor car industry is geared to the concept of rapid production and rapid consumption: cars are not built to last and within a short time they are replaced by new models. Old cars 'decompose' and little of the steel is re-cycled and used to make new cars. If it were re-cycled there would not be the same demand for iron ore and the economy of the pro-ducer countries would suffer. On the other hand there is clearly a limit to the available resources of new iron ore and the time will come when re-cycling is a necessity. It would also be technically possible to manufacture cars that last a long time. This would be less demanding on the dwindling raw materials (including many in addition to iron) but would presumably create unemployment for car workers in Britain and miners in Africa, and would reduce the profits made by business and by the government. It would also mean a change in the social attitudes of people in developed coun-tries who would have to buy one car to last a lifetime rather than replace the car with a new model at the first opportunity. Steel is also used in construction work and thus becomes 'locked up' for long periods of time, chiefly in the developed countries where most construction occurs. This pattern of production and consumption applies to all other non-renewable resources, many of them produced by under-developed countries, and all of them consumed mainly by developed countries.

The most significant aspect of the above considerations is that the present economic structure of the world would collapse if the developed countries were unable to use the resources of the under-developed countries. This is most strikingly apparent with oil which is produced mostly in under-developed countries (although not a great quantity is produced in tropical Africa) and consumed largely in developed countries. It is equally significant that there would be economic collapse if the under-developed countries consumed raw materials at the same rate as the developed countries.

The present concern of the industrial countries with the harmful effects of environmental pollution is regarded as something of a threat to development by the under-developed countries. Cleaner industry and more re-cycling of raw materials, both of which are now being advocated in industrial countries, could easily make industrialization a more expensive process, and this might inhibit rather than promote development in Africa. It has been suggested that if the industrial countries are worried about the effects of pollution there should be an effort to spread industry out on a global

THE ECOLOGY OF DEVELOPMENT 181

basis: many people in tropical Africa would welcome the sight of chimneys belching smoke as this is equated with development and jobs. There is much to be said in favour of this point of view but there seems little prospect of it being implemented.

The present ecological predicament in tropical Africa can be defined in relatively simple terms. Human numbers are expanding extremely rapidly as a result of the decreased death rate among children. The decrease has been brought about by the suppression (to a large extent) of the effects of many of the important killing diseases and by the spread of cultivation. Everywhere there are understandable demands for a higher standard of living which in effect means a higher rate of consumption of raw materials. All plans for economic development are in one way or another intended to facilitate a better standard of living which in Africa, unless there is a radical change in attitude, will result in even higher rates of population increase. The increase in human numbers in Africa has taken place chiefly in the last few hundred years and is continuing at an accelerating pace. The savanna and forest ecosystems which have taken thousands of years to evolve their biological complexity and stability have been largely destroyed, and almost everywhere there are signs of cultivation, erosion, and a general degradation of the environment. Raw materials have been exploited and exploitation is continuing, chiefly to the benefit of the developed countries. The population is largely dependent on food that it can produce for itself and the food that it can acquire from other countries in exchange for raw materials or in the form of aid. There is virtually no industry and prospects for industrial development seem poor. Indeed even if industrialization were possible it could proceed little further than producing goods for home consumption as the developed nations are unlikely to require quantities of manufactured goods from Africa. This predicament is not of course unique to Africa: it applies to varying extents to almost all tropical countries, and the paradox is that the continued existence of developed countries is dependent on this unsatisfactory state of affairs.

Table 27 shows the world population in 1960 and the projected population in 1980 and 2000. The projections are based on estimated current birth and death rates and are therefore optimistic as it is assumed that there will be no rise in the rate of population increase.

Other estimates give higher and lower figures for 1980 and 2000, depending on what assumptions are made about fertility trends and death rates. The figures in Table 27 are divided into regions and these in turn are divided into developed and under-developed areas of the world. Almost all the under-developed areas are in the tropics. As indicated in Chapter 2, there is much disagreement among economists as to what is meant by development and under-development, indeed doubt has been expressed as to whether it is legitimate to consider development in economic terms. Economists consider that literacy, income per head (which in effect means the capacity to consume raw materials), child mortality rates, housing, and so on, can be used to judge the degree of economic development in a country, but all of these present numerous difficulties of interpretation. How can one say, for instance, that a country that grows most of its own food and yet has a low *per capita* income is less developed than one with a higher *per capita* income which has to import most of its food? In Table 27 development is defined in demographic terms: an under-developed country has a rate of population increase that is known or believed to be in excess of 2 per cent per year, while a developed country has a population growth rate of less than this figure. By adopting this definition it is assumed that the rate of population increase is the chief obstacle to economic improvement in an under-developed country, but the definition evades the question of whether economic improvement is necessarily a good thing or for how long the present inequality among the countries of the world can be sustained.

The projected figures in Table 27 show that although the present population of Africa (including that of the area outside the tropics) is lower than that of Europe, it should become equal to that of Europe some time in the 1980s, and by the year 2000 there may be nearly 300 million more people in Africa than in Europe. The ecological impact of this projected rise in human numbers will be spectacular. Moreover the estimate of 300 million more may be on the conservative side. Thus recent reports from Rhodesia indicate that the African population is increasing at a rate of 3·6 per cent per year which means that the population will double itself in about eighteen years, a phenomenon which will have political as well as economic implications.

15 The Library, University of Ghana. Many of the universities in tropical Africa are well equipped and offer a comprehensive range of courses for students at all levels. Some African universities are academically superior to many of those in developed countries.

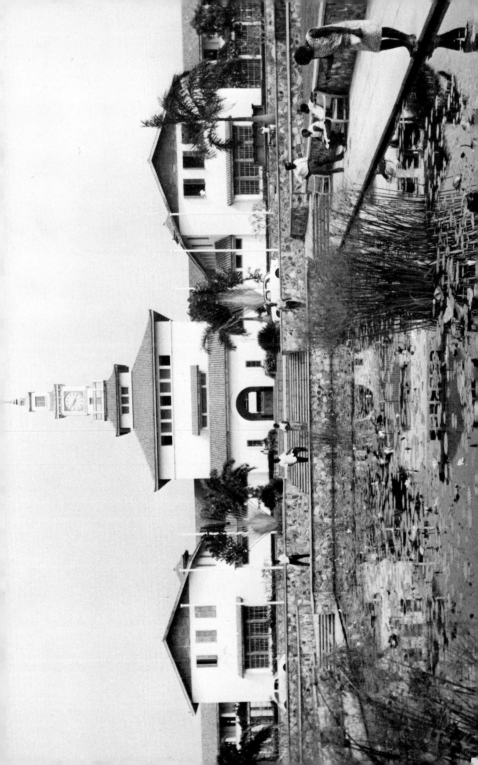

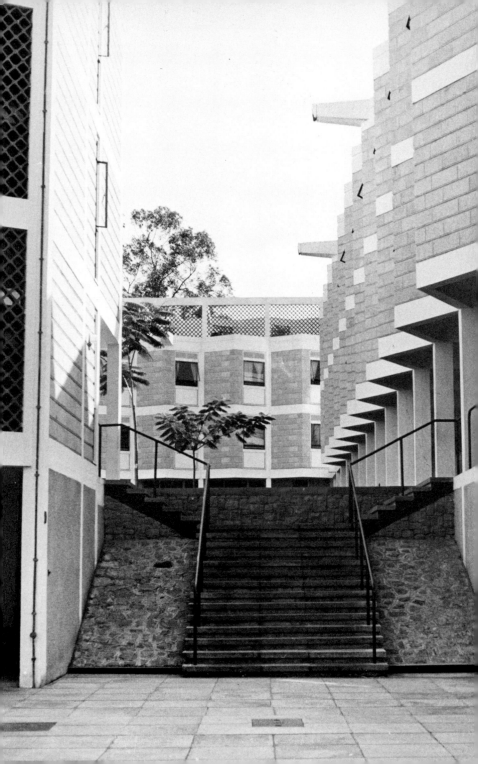

Most African countries are forced by circumstances to encourage economic investment from the developed countries. Some people see this as a form of aid but in reality it amounts to little more than a financial inducement for Africa to export more of its natural resources and to accept in return manufactured products from the developed countries. The motives of the European, American, Russian, and Chinese governments in offering aid to the newly independent nations of Africa are not so much associated with making profits but with gaining influence, which, of course, in time, can lead to making profits. The former colonial powers probably feel somewhat guilty about what they did not do in the past or they are embarrassed because they failed to predict the unexpected turns that political events have taken. There is also the curious view that Africans need help and advice more than other people which in its extreme form can lead to disastrous situations where anything African must not be criticized. This does no good, and it is important to appreciate that Africans, like other people, can make mistakes and can become corrupted, a point which is expanded at considerable length by Andreski (1968). But perhaps the most important motive in offering aid is the possibility of political influence. Whether in fact there is any long-term influence is another matter, but the big powers evidently feel that there is some advantage to be gained if they can claim support for their international policies from under-developed countries. The present declining influence of the United Nations in determining world events will perhaps result in a decrease in aid for entirely political purposes; indeed there may be an increase in bilateral aid more closely associated with marketing and economic development.

It is probably true to say that since the days of independence no area in the world has suffered at the hands of outside experts more than tropical Africa. There are experts in education from UNESCO, in agriculture from FAO, in health from WHO; there are those that give advice on economic development, how to build airports, roads, universities, and television centres, and those that want to try and preserve wildlife and areas of land which they claim are of scientific and aesthetic interest to the rest of the world. All are anxious to offer advice and to propose programmes which, they urge, are related to development and to the well-being of the people. Individual

16 Student halls of residence at Makerere University, Uganda. Students at African universities enjoy excellent working facilities, but it is a pity that once qualified so few of them are prepared to teach in the schools in the more remote rural areas.

proposals may conflict and rivalries often develop between organizations trying to achieve the same ends. Africa is remarkably receptive to the ideas of others and missionaries have for years exploited this, but the missionaries now have to compete with the economists, educationists, and conservationists for the attention of the people. But the advent of the expert into African society does not appear to have achieved a great deal. There are probably a number of reasons for this, not the least of which is that many experts are badly informed, not only on the subject they are supposed to know something about, but also on the environment on which the organization they represent wishes to make an impact. This applies especially to the experts from the specialized agencies of the United Nations who are often appointed to their highly paid jobs for political reasons (each member state is entitled to contribute its quota of experts) rather than because of their abilities in a particular field. Then there is the problem of implementation. African politicians are often more than willing to receive offers of assistance for their country, especially if there are no strings attached, but if it becomes necessary that the recipient country should also contribute money and manpower to a scheme, difficulties arise, and in many cases little or nothing is achieved. But the chief difficulty with outside offers of assistance is that only rarely are the long-term effects of a proposal evaluated. Thus a short-term proposal to eradicate a disease or to improve crop production very often leads to little more than a local increase in population.

In the developed countries there are numerous charitable organizations whose aim is to relieve hunger, malnutrition, and the effects of disease, and to improve the agriculture. Their funds are dispersed in so many different projects that virtually all their efforts are short-term. OXFAM is one of the best known of the charitable organizations and (to take an example) in the year beginning in October 1965 it allocated about £385 000 to about 170 projects in 22 tropical African countries. About a third of the money was allocated to projects aimed at preventing disease and another third to projects associated with improving food production. Just over 8 per cent was allocated to help victims of civil wars and to feed refugees, most of whom had fled from one independent country to another. About 22 per cent was allocated to training programmes, mostly associated with rural health and agriculture, but only 1·2 per cent went to family planning, the one project that might be expected to have more than short-term benefits. Indeed in the year in question there were only two allocations under this heading, one to Kenya and one to Sierra Leone, and the total amount granted was only £4743.

Most of the people of tropical Africa are illiterate and with expanding human populations there seems little possibility that literacy will become widespread in the immediate future. There are campaigns aimed at providing more schools and offering facilities for adults to become literate but most efforts are frustrated by the rise in the population. Many of the existing schools, especially those in rural areas, are staffed by incompetent teachers, many of them expatriates from Europe, America, and India. One difficulty is in persuading African graduates from the universities to take up teaching as a career. Most students receiving diplomas and degrees look towards the civil service (or its equivalent) or to business enterprises for jobs which not only offer a better salary and allowances but also carry more status. School teaching is often regarded as a last resort, to be entertained only as a temporary measure until something better comes along. There are, of course, some dedicated teachers, but many teach only because they have failed elsewhere, and it is likely that the continuing recruitment of teachers from abroad is preventing a development of local interest in teaching as a profession.

The universities of tropical Africa have developed much more rapidly than the schools. In most countries there are well-equipped universities that not only provide instruction to a high standard, but are also actively involved in research. Most of the scientific research is of an applied nature, but there is some pure research, which is sometimes criticized by politicians as not being relevant to national development. Several African academics have argued persuasively that there is a place for pure research as it trains people in the art of problem solving and exercises the imagination. It has been said that university facilities have developed too quickly, especially in relation to the situation in the schools, but on the other hand a big expansion of school education, especially at the elementary level, would lead to the production of large numbers of semi-literate people for whom there are no jobs. Illiteracy may be a big problem, but large numbers of literate people could create a bigger one in the present environment.

Earlier in this book it has been suggested that improving the agriculture and eradicating disease will not in themselves result in a significant improvement in the already unsatisfactory state of affairs. The agricultural experts in particular have misled Africa into believing that the solution to poverty is to grow more food. More food for what? one might ask. It does not matter whether agriculture becomes highly mechanized or whether the approach urged by Dumont (1966), in which the silent majority (the peasant farmers) make an all-out effort to grow more food by using relatively simple methods, is adopted, the result will be the same: more people. The so-called 'green revolution', invented by the western countries, but also practised by the eastern countries, is a myth, although without doubt big business will benefit from the increased sales of pesticides, fertilizers, and improved varieties of crops.

Prospects and possibilities for industrial development in Africa on the scale that has been possible in Europe, America, and Japan are remote: the industrial nations already have all the advantages in the highly competitive world of commerce and industry, and it is unrealistic to suppose that there will be a change in this position. It is to me inconceivable that a tropical African nation will be able to develop its industry sufficiently to produce and sell items like motor cars and jet aircraft to the industrial nations or even in competition with them. There is perhaps a little hope if the African nations can offer items or services for sale that are impossible to obtain elsewhere. It is not easy to imagine what many of these might be, but one obvious one is tourism. In East Africa in particular there are numerous tourist attractions, including game parks, which if developed further could produce a substantial revenue, and the same applies to the numerous attractive beaches which are much sought after by sun-loving Europeans with money to spend. The advantage of tourism is that it offers something that cannot be had elsewhere and, moreover, it does not result in a flow of raw materials out of the country. The packaging and marketing of crop products instead of exporting them as raw materials also comes to mind, but many of these crops are also grown elsewhere in the tropics, a possible exception being cocoa, most of the world's supply coming from a few countries in West Africa. Would it be possible for the cocoa-growing countries to stop exporting the raw product and to develop industries that result in marketing the finished products? But these and similar possibilities will do no more than merely scratch the surface of the problem. None is likely to produce the effect that everyone is hoping for: an expanding economy and a rapidly rising standard of living for the people.

The theme of this book has been man's struggle to exist in a complex tropical environment. Economic development in Africa is impeded by the phenomenal growth of the human population and by the necessity, imposed by the industrial nations of the world, for Africa to function as a producer of raw materials for consumption elsewhere. If there is to be a solution to the present predicament there must be a massive effort to slow down the rate of population growth and a policy on the part of the industrial nations to de-develop sufficiently to allow under-developed countries to catch up. Neither of these stands much chance of being implemented in the immediate future. Sustained economic growth is the goal of all governments, both left and right wing, in both developed and under-developed countries, and although a diverse array of people have come to realize that in order to survive growth must be controlled, there is at the moment no political party in the world that would adopt this as its manifesto and expect to come to power by either democratic or other means.

TABLES

TABLE I

Estimated population and population density of tropical African countries. The figures refer to the mid-sixties. Offshore islands are excluded. Based on figures given in the U.N. Demographic Yearbook for 1965.

	Area in thousands km²	Estimated population (thousands)	Density km²	Annual rate of increase %
Senegal	196	3 400	17	2·3
The Gambia	11	324	29	2·4
Portuguese Guinea	36	525	15	0·2
Guinea	246	3 420	14	2·8
Mali	1 201	4 485	4	2·3
Sierra Leone	72	2 240	31	2·1
Liberia	111	1 041	9	1·4
Ivory Coast	322	3 750	12	3·3
Upper Volta	274	4 750	17	2·5
Ghana	239	7 537	32	2·7
Togo	57	1 603	28	2·8
Dahomey	113	2 300	20	2·9
Niger	1 267	3 237	3	3·3
Nigeria	924	56 400	61	2·0
Cameroon	475	5 103	11	2·1
Equatorial Guinea	28	263	9	1·9
Gabon	268	459	2	1·6
Congo Brazzaville	342	826	2	1·6
Congo Kinshasa	2 345	15 300	7	2·1
Angola	1 247	5 084	4	1·4
Central African Republic	623	1 320	2	2·2
Chad	1 284	3 300	3	1·5
Zambia	753	3 600	5	2·9
Rhodesia	389	4 140	11	3·3
Mozambique	783	6 872	9	1·3
Malawi	119	3 900	33	2·8
Tanzania	937	9 990	11	1·9
Burundi	28	3 000	101	2·5
Rwanda	26	3 018	115	3·1
Uganda	236	7 367	31	2·5
Kenya	583	9 104	16	2·9
Sudan	2 506	13 180	5	2·8
Ethiopia	1 222	22 200	18	1·8
Somali Republic	638	2 420	4	3·5
Total	19 901	215 458		

NOTE: The present (1972) population is probably considerably higher than the figures shown above, and in some countries there may already be nearly half as many people again as the figures shown.

TABLE 2 *Income per head in 1962 in some tropical African countries. From Hodder (1968).*

	Income per head in U.S. dollars		Income per head in U.S. dollars
Senegal	44	Gabon	72
The Gambia	46	Congo Brazzaville	50
Portuguese Guinea	40	Congo Kinshasa	67
Guinea	39	Angola	52
Mali	37	Central African	
Sierra Leone	47	Republic	41
Liberia	43	Chad	39
Ivory Coast	89	Zambia	96
Upper Volta	39	Rhodesia	156
Ghana	179	Mozambique	42
Togo	44	Malawi	49
Dahomey	49	Tanzania	50
Niger	36	Burundi	29
Nigeria	66	Rwanda	40
Cameroon	50	Uganda	57
Equatorial Guinea	49	Kenya	72

TABLE 3 *Birth and death rates and expectation of life at birth in some tropical African countries. From U.N. Demographic Yearbook for 1965.*

	Birth rate per thousand	Death rate per thousand	Infant death rate per thousand	Expectation of life at birth Males	Females
Senegal	43	17	93		
The Gambia	39	21			
Guinea	62	40	216	26	28
Mali	61	30	123		
Ivory Coast	56	33			
Upper Volta	50	32	182	32	31
Ghana	47–52	24	156	—38—	
Togo	55	29	127	32	39
Dahomey	54	26	111	—37—	
Niger	52	27	200		
Gabon	35	30	229	25	45
Congo Brazzaville	41	24	180	—37—	
Congo Kinshasa	43	20	104	38	40
Central African Rep.	48	30	190	33	36
Chad	46	31	165	—30—	
Zambia	51	20	259	—40—	
Rhodesia	48	14	122	—50—	
Tanzania	46	25	190	—35-40—	
Burundi	47	17	121		
Rwanda	52	14	137		
Uganda	42	20	160		
Kenya	50	20		—40-45—	
Sudan	52	19	94		

TABLE 4

Intervals between births at Imesi, Nigeria. From Martin et al. (1964).

	Number of births	9-11	12-17	18-23	24-29	30-35	36-41	42-47	48+	Mean
					Months between births					
Following survival of preceding child	248	—	1	9	24	127	52	20	15	36
Following stillbirth or death of child in first year	34	10	14	5	3	1	—	—	1	17

TABLE 5

Comparison of interval between births (in months) with the survival of the preceding child at Imesi, Nigeria, and Cocos-Keeling, South Pacific. From Martin et al. (1964).

	Number of births	1	2	3	4	5	6	7+	Mean
		Birth order of preceding child							
Imesi	248	32	35	36	36	34	38	38	35·5
Cocos-Keeling	1692	26	29	29	31	32	31	30	29·4

TABLE 6

Seasonal variation in the frequency of twin births in a Nigerian village. From Knox and Morley (1960).

	Twins	Single births	% Twins
January	6	196	3·0
February	12	191	5·9
March	9	196	4·4
April	10	218	4·4
May	17	124	7·4
June	11	208	5·0
July	17	153	6·3
August	17	199	7·9
September	15	247	5·7
October	19	290	6·2
November	14	321	4·2
December	11	281	3·8

TABLE 7

Ethnic composition (per cent) of the population of Sierra Leone in 1963.
From Clarke (1966).

Creoles	1·9	Loko	2·9
Fula	3·1	Mandingo	2·3
Gallinas	0·1	Mende	30·9
Gola	0·2	Sherbro	3·4
Kissi	2·3	Susu	3·1
Kono	4·8	Temne	29·8
Koranko	3·7	Vai	0·3
Krim	0·4	Yalunka	0·7
Kru	0·2	No tribe	1·3
Limba	8·4	Others	0·2

TABLE 8

The age structure of the population of Sierra Leone in 1963.
From Clarke (1966).

	Number	%		Number	%
under 5	377 335	17·3	35–39	136 384	6·3
5–9	280 649	12·9	40–44	114 758	5·3
10–14	142 420	6·5	45–49	85 531	3·9
15–19	194 378	8·9	50–54	69 957	3·2
20–24	190 784	8·7	55–59	41 760	1·9
25–29	207 753	9·5	60–64	55 954	2·6
30–34	172 183	7·9	65 and over	110 509	5·1

TABLE 9

Sex ratio by age in the population of Sierra Leone in 1963.
From Clarke (1966).

	Females per thousand males		Females per thousand males
under 5	1014	35–39	882
5–9	928	40–44	822
10–14	874	45–49	714
15–19	1346	50–54	763
20–24	1526	55–59	729
25–29	1221	60–64	857
30–34	1106	65 and over	868

TABLE 10

Common diseases in 95 babies at Sukuta, The Gambia, during their first 18 months of life. From Marsden (1964).

	Number of attacks recorded	% of babies affected
Conjunctivitis	143	73
Upper respiratory infections	122	76
Lower respiratory infections	89	59
Diarrhoea	88	55
Skin sores	78	51
Cracks behind ears	66	42
Insect bites	64	50
Malaria requiring treatment	59	46
Abscesses and boils	46	34
Otitis media	42	26
Prickly heat	30	26
Thrush	22	20
Measles	21	22
Overt malnutrition	18	14
Fungus infections of skin	16	16
Scabies	12	10
Whooping cough	11	11

TABLE 11

Deaths of children under 10 years of age caused by measles in Keneba and Jali, The Gambia, 12 February–24 April 1961. Adapted from McGregor (1964).

Age in months	Number of children	Deaths	% mortality
0–6	42	3	7·1
7–12	39	12	30·8
13–24	64	16	25·0
25–36	35	10	28·6
37–48	42	10	23·8
49–60	37	5	13·5
61–72	42	1	2·4
73–84	40	0	—
85–96	29	0	—
97–108	34	4	11·8
109–120	33	1	3·0
Total	437	62	14·2

TABLE 12

Monthly distribution of deaths in children under five years of age at Jali, The Gambia, in 1957–63. Stillbirths are excluded. From McGregor (1964).

Year	Jan.	Feb.	Mar.	Apr.	May	Jun.	Jul.	Aug.	Sep.	Oct.	Nov.	Dec.	Unknown	Total
1957	—	—	—	—	1	—	—	2	3	2	—	2	—	10
1958	—	1	—	2	3	—	2	4	1	1	1	2	1	18
1959	2	—	—	—	1	—	—	2	1	—	2	1	1	10
1960	3	2	—	—	—	—	—	—	2	2	1	2	—	12
1961	—	3	15	7	1	—	—	2	—	1	1	—	—	30
1962	1	—	1	2	—	—	2	2	4	6	6	4	1	29
1963	1	—	2	2	—	—	—	1	5	2	7	2	—	22
Total	7	6	18	13	6	—	4	13	16	14	18	13	3	131

TABLE 13

Average age at which children suffer from measles and whooping cough in different parts of the world. Adapted from Morley (1967).

	Measles		Whooping cough	
	Number of cases	Average age in months	Number of cases	Average age in months
West Africa	17 580	20	2 569	24
East Africa	5 798	23	2 778	35
Congo and South Africa	2 198	29	860	24
Jordan	2 038	18	942	24
Lebanon and North Africa	422	31	554	36
England and Wales	306 721	53	92 266	46
Massachusetts			7 445	62

TABLE 14

Frequency of diseases in a sample of 170 migrant labourers and 599 other inhabitants at Jimma, Ethiopia. From Giel and Van Luijk (1967).

	% Labourers	Others
Malaria	16·5	6·3
Venereal diseases	12·9	2·0
Fevers of unknown origin	12·9	6·7
Neglected wounds and ulcers	10·6	2·3
Dysentery	4·7	3·1
Tuberculosis	4·7	2·3
Pneumonia	2·9	2·8
Relapsing fever	2·3	0·6
Severe malnutrition	1·7	2·3
Leprosy	1·7	0·2 (1 case)
Hepatitis	1·7	0·4
Schistosomiasis	1·7	0·4
Onchocerciasis	0·5 (1 case)	0·4

TABLE 15

Ethnic composition and place of birth of people in a mining area (Lunsar, Sierra Leone) and in the surrounding rural villages. From Mills (1967a).

	% Lunsar	Rural villages
Temne	76·2	93·8
Mende	2·3	0·5
Fula	5·1	1·4
Limba	7·1	1·1
Creole	1·6	—
others	7·7	3·3
Born locally	28·8	71·1

TABLE 16

Comparison of morbidity rates in Lunsar, Sierre Leone, a mining town, and in the surrounding rural villages. From Mills (1967a).

	% positive for Malaria	Onchocerciasis	Nutritional deficiency
Lunsar	78·2	49·5	16·8
Villages	93·5	47·0	74·8

TABLE 17

Some features of phases in desert locusts. From Uvarov (1961b).

	Phase *solitaria*	Phase *gregaria*
Behaviour		
Tendency to aggregate	absent	present
Mobility	low	high
Activity rhythm	not synchronized	synchronized
Adult flight	nocturnal	diurnal
Physiology		
Food and water reserves at birth	lower	higher
Early mortality of young	higher	lower
Development rate	slower	faster
Instar number	greater	less
Fecundity	more, but smaller eggs	fewer, but larger eggs
Coloration		
Hopper coloration	uniform green	yellow-black pattern
Adult coloration	no changes	changes with maturation and age
Morphology		
Head	smaller	larger
Tegmen	shorter	longer
Hind femur	longer	shorter
Sexual size dimorphism	pronounced	slight

TABLE 18

Frequency (per cent) of the three main grass components in the diets of the wildebeest, topi, and zebra. From Gwynne and Bell (1968).

	Dry season			Wet season	
Grass part	Wildebeest	Topi	Zebra	Wildebeest	Zebra
leaf	17·2	9·4	0·2	61·3	36·8
sheath	52·7	53·4	48·7	28·9	43·9
stem	30·1	37·2	51·0	8·0	15·0

The zebra also eats small quantities of dicotyledon leaf in the dry season and some grass seeds in the wet season. The wildebeest eats small quantities of dicotyledons in the wet season.

TABLE 19

Approximate protein content of some common foods. From Arthur (1969).

	% Protein (fresh weight)	% Protein (dry weight)
cassava	0·9	2·4
maize	9·2	10·5
rice (milled)	7·6	8·7
spinach	2·3	29·1
beans	22·1	25·0
beef	18·5	48·7
chicken	20·2	59·4
eggs	12·8	49·2
fish	18·8	72·6
milk	3·5	27·6

TABLE 20

Blood loss in relation to number of Schistosoma haematobium eggs in the urine. From Jordan (1961).

Number of cases	Eggs per 10 ml of urine	Average blood loss in mm³ per litre of urine
41	1–20	3
33	21–60	29
19	61–120	42
9	121–200	178
8	201–350	850
6	351–1500	2733

TABLE 21

Effect of age on incidence of Schistosoma haematobium infection among people in a village in Tanzania and average number of eggs in urine. From Jordan (1961).

Age-group in years	Number examined	% Positive	Average egg density in 10 ml of urine
0–5	86	24	34
6–12	106	78	64
13–20	61	74	17
21–30	85	54	13
31–40	42	48	9
41–50	25	68	6
51–60	33	55	11
over 60	13	54	4

TABLE 22

Results of treating Asian schoolboys with Astiban as a cure for schistosomiasis. From Bell (1964).

	Number treated	Number cured
Vegetarians	11	1
Non-vegetarians	25	13

TABLE 23

Mean number of erupted teeth in children at given ages. From McGregor, Thomson, and Billewicz (1968).

Age in months	U.S.A.	London	Paris	Zürich	Dakar	The Gambia
6	0·4	0·4	0·4	0·4		0·3
9	3·1	2·8	2·9	2·5	2·7	2·2
12	5·9	6·1	5·8	5·4	4·7	4·5
18	12·4	12·9	12·3	12·2	11·4	10·9
24	16·7	16·3	16·4	16·3	16·4	17·4
36	19·9	20·0				20·0

TABLE 24

The frequency of red–green colour blindness among male Africans from different ages and of different ethnic groups. From Roberts (1967).

Locality	People	Number tested	% red–green colour blind
Uganda	Baganda	537	1·86
Congo	Congo Bantu	929	1·72
Rwanda and Burundi	Bahutu	1000	2·70
	Batutsi	1000	2·56
Nigeria	Habe	368	1·90
	Fulani	178	1·69
	Other Hausa	63	1·59
	Yoruba	60	3·37
	Ogoni	239	2·09
	Abua	141	2·13
Tanzania	Hangaza and Bushubi	123	1·63
Kenya	'Bantu'	198	2·46

TABLE 25

Gene flow rates in three groups of Nilotic people. From Roberts (1965).

Recipient population	Donating population		
	Nuer	Dinka	Shilluk
Nuer	0·9850	0·0125	0·0025
Dinka	0·0138	0·9775	0·0087
Shilluk	0	0·0098	0·9902

TABLE 26

Accumulated admixture in three groups of Nilotic people after twenty generations. From Roberts (1965).

Recipient population	Donating population		
	Nuer	Dinka	Shilluk
Nuer	0·7637	0·1810	0·0553
Dinka	0·1961	0·6693	0·1346
Shilluk	0·0195	0·1465	0·8340

TABLE 27

Present and projected population of the world in millions. From Taylor (1969).

	1960	1980	2000
World	2998	4519	7522
Developed	976	1242	1580
Under-developed	2022	3277	5942
Regional estimates			
Developed			
Europe	425	496	571
U.S.S.R.	214	295	402
North America	199	272	388
Japan	93	114	127
Temperate South America	33	47	68
Oceania	16	22	33
Under-developed			
Mainland East Asia	654	942	1509
Remainder of East Asia	47	87	175
South Asia	865	1446	2702
Africa	273	458	860
Latin America (part)	180	340	688

BIBLIOGRAPHY

ALBRECHT, F. O. (1962) Some physiological and ecological aspects of locust phases. *Trans. R. ent. Soc. Lond.*, 114:335–75.

ALLAN, W. (1965) *The African husbandman.* Oliver and Boyd, Edinburgh and London.

ALLISON, A. C. (1954a) The distribution of the sickle-cell trait in East Africa and elsewhere, and its apparent relationship to the incidence of subtertian malaria. *Trans. R. Soc. trop. Med. Hyg.*, 48:312–18.

(1954b) Protection by the sickle-cell trait against subtertian malarial infection. *B. med. J.*, 1:290–4.

(1954c) Notes on sickle-cell polymorphism. *Ann. hum. Genet.*, 19:39–57.

(1969) Natural selection and population diversity. *J. biosoc. Sci. Suppl.*, 1:15–30.

ANDRESKI, S. (1968) *The African predicament. A study in the pathology of modernisation.* Michael Joseph, London.

ARTHUR, D. R. (1969) *Survival. Man and his environment.* English Universities Press, London.

ASHCROFT, M. T. (1959) The importance of African wild animals as reservoirs of trypanosomiasis. *E. Afr. med. J.*, 36:3–11.

BALFOUR-BROWNE, F. L. (1960) The green muscardine disease of insects, with special reference to an epidemic in a swarm of locusts in Eritrea. *Proc. R. ent. Soc. Lond.* A, 35:65–74.

BATTEN, A. (1967) Seasonal movements of swarms of *Locusta migratoria migratorioides* (R. & F.) in western Africa from 1928 to 1931. *Bull. ent. Res.*, 57:357–80.

(1969) The Senegalese grasshopper *Oedaleus senegalensis* Krauss. *J. appl. Ecol.*, 6:27–45.

BELL, D. R. (1964) Diet and therapy in Bilharzia. *Lancet*, 1:643–4.

BESS, H. A. (1964) Populations of the leaf-miner *Leucoptera meyricki* Ghesq. and its parasites in sprayed and unsprayed coffee in Kenya. *Bull. ent. Res.*, 55:59–82.

BLUM, H. F. (1961) Does the melanin pigment of human skin have adaptive value? An essay in human ecology and the evolution of race. *Q. Rev. Biol.*, 36:50–63.

BODENHEIMER, F. S. (1951) *Insects as human food.* Junk, The Hague.

BOTHA, D. H. (1967) Some phase characteristics of the southern African form of the desert locust (*Schistocerca gregaria* (Forskål)). *S. Afr. J. agric. Sci.*, 10:61–76.

BRASS, W., COALE, A. J., DEMENY, P., HEISEL, D. F., LORIMER, F., ROMANUIK, A., and VAN DE WALLE, E. (1968) *The demography of tropical Africa.* Princeton University Press, Princeton, New Jersey.

BURKITT, D. (1958) A sarcoma involving the jaw in African children. *B. J. Surg.*, 46:218–23.

CARLISLE, D. B., ELLIS, P. E., and BETTS, E. (1965) The influence of aromatic shrubs on sexual maturation in the desert locust *Schistocerca gregaria*. *J. Insect Physiol.*, 11:1541–58.

CARLISLE, D. B., ELLIS, P. E., and OSBORNE, D. J. (1969) Effects of plant growth regulators on locusts and cotton stainer bugs. *J. Sci. Fd. Agric.*, 20:391–3.

CARR-SAUNDERS, A. M. (1922) *The population problem: a study in human evolution*. Clarendon Press, Oxford.

CHAPMAN, W. M. (1965) Ocean science and human protein malnutrition problems in middle Africa. *Inst. Int. Stud. Univ. Calif. Res. Ser.*, 9:161–84.

CLARK, J. D. (1951) *The prehistory of southern Africa*. Penguin Books, London.
    (1960) Human ecology during Pleistocene and later times in Africa south of the Sahara. *Curr. Anthrop.*, 1:307–24.
    (1964) The prehistoric origins of African agriculture. *J. Afr. Hist.*, 5:161–83.

CLARKE, C. A. (1970) *Human genetics and medicine*. Arnold, London.

CLARKE, J. I. (ed.) (1966) *Sierra Leone in maps*. University of London Press, London.

COBLEY, L. S. (1956) *An introduction to the botany of tropical crops*. Longmans, London.

COKER, W. Z. (1966) Linkage of the DDT-resistant gene in some strains of *Aedes aegypti* (L.). *Ann. trop. Med. Parasit.*, 60:347–56.

COLE, S. (1963) *Races of man*. British Museum (Natural History), London.

CORBET, P. S. (1964) Observations on mosquitoes ovipositing in small containers in Zika Forest, Uganda. *J. anim. Ecol.*, 33:141–64.

CROWE, T. J. (1964) Coffee leaf miners in Kenya. *Kenya Coffee*, June 1964:1–5.

CROWE, T. J., and LEEUWANGH, J. (1965) The green looper. *Kenya Coffee*, Oct. 1965:1–4.

DALZIEL, J. M. (1937) *The useful plants of west tropical Africa*. Crown Agents, London.

DAVIDSON, A. (1963) Insects attacking *Striga* in Kenya. *Nature, Lond.*, 197:923.

DAVIES, H. (1967) *Tsetse flies in Northern Nigeria*. Ibadan University Press, Ibadan.

DAVIES, J. C., and GREATHEAD, D. J. (1967) Occurrence of *Teleonemia scrupulosa* on *Sesamum indicum* Linn. in Uganda. *Nature, Lond.*, 213:102–3.

DEAN, G. J. W. (1967) Observations on the structure of hopper bands and movements of hoppers of the red locust (*Nomadacris septemfasciatus* Serville). *J. ent. Soc. sth Afr.*, 30:1–17.

DUKE, B. O. L., LEWIS, D. J., and MOORE, P. J. (1966) *Onchocerca-Simulium* complexes. I. Transmission of forest and Sudan-savanna strains of *Onchocerca volvulus*, from Cameroon, by *Simulium damnosum* from various West African bioclimatic zones. *Ann. trop. Med. Parasit.*, 60:318–36.

DUKE, B. O. L., and MOORE, P. J. (1968) The contribution of different age groups to the transmission of onchocerciasis in a Cameroon forest village. *Trans. R. Soc. trop. Med. Hyg.*, 62:22–8.

DUMONT, R. (1966) *False start in Africa*. Deutsch, London.

DUNN, J. A. (1963) Insecticide resistance in the cocoa capsid, *Distantiella theobroma* (Dist.). *Nature, Lond.*, 199:1207.

EKPECHI, O. L., DIMITRIADOU, A., and FRASER, R. (1966) Goitrogenic activity of cassava (a staple Nigerian food). *Nature, Lond.*, 210:1137–8.

ELLIS, P. (1968) Can insect hormones and their mimics be used to control pests? *PANS*, 14:329–42.

ELLIS, P. E., CARLISLE, D. B., and OSBORNE, D. J. (1965) Desert locusts: sexual maturation delayed by feeding on senescent vegetation. *Science, N.Y.*, 149:546–7.

ENTWISTLE, P. F. (ed.) (1964) *Proceedings of the conference on mirids and other pests of cocoa*. West African Cocoa Research Institute, Ibadan.

FISHER, R. A. (1930) *The genetical theory of natural selection*. Clarendon Press, Oxford.

FORBES, C. D., MACKAY, N., and KHAN, A. A. (1966) Christmas disease and haemophilia in Kenya. *Trans. R. Soc. trop. Med. Hyg.*, 60:777–81.

FORD, E. B. (1965) *Genetic polymorphism*. Faber and Faber, London.

FOSTER, R. (1967a) Schistosomiasis on an irrigated estate in East Africa. I. The background. *J. trop. Med. Hyg.*, 70:133–40.

(1967b) Schistosomiasis on an irrigated estate in East Africa. II. Epidemiology. *J. trop. Med. Hyg.*, 70:159–68.

(1967c) Schistosomiasis on an irrigated estate in East Africa. III. Effects of asymptomatic infection on health and industrial efficiency. *J. trop. Med. Hyg.*, 70:185–95.

GARNHAM, P. C. C. (1966) *Malaria parasites and other Haemosporidia*. Blackwell, Oxford.

GEIER, P. W. (1966) Management of insect pests. *A. Rev. Ent.*, 11:471–90.

GERLACH, L. P. (1965) Nutrition in its sociocultural matrix: food getting and using along the East African coast. *Inst. Int. Stud. Univ. Calif. Res. Ser.*, 9:245–68.

GIEL, R., and VAN LUIJK, J. N. (1967) The plight of the daily labourer in a coffee growing province of Ethiopia. *Trop. geogrl. Med.*, 19:304–8.

GIGLIOLI, M. E. C. (1965) Some observations on blister beetles, family Meloidae, in Gambia, West Africa. *Trans. R. Soc. trop. Med. Hyg.*, 59:657–63.

GILLES, H. M., and MCGREGOR, I. A. (1961) Studies on the significance of high serum gamma-globulin concentrations in Gambian Africans. III. Gamma-globulin concentrations in Gambian women protected from malaria for two years. *Ann. trop. Med. Parasit.*, 55:463–7.

GILLIES, M. T., and SMITH, A. (1960) The effect of a residual house-spraying campaign in East Africa on species balance in the *Anopheles funestus* group. The replacement of *A. funestus* Giles by *A. rivulorum* Leeson. *Bull. ent. Res.*, 51:243–52.

GLASGOW, J. P. (1963) *The distribution and abundance of tsetse*. Pergamon, London.

GLOVER, P. E. (1965) A review of recent knowledge of the relationship between the tsetse fly and its vertebrate hosts. *IUCN Publ. New Series*, 6:1–84.

GLOVER, P. E., TRUMP, E. C., and WATERIDGE, L. E. D. (1964) Termitaria and vegetation patterns on the Loita plains of Kenya. *J. Ecol.*, 52:367–77.

GOMA, L. K. H. (1961) The influence of man's activities on swamp breeding mosquitoes in Uganda (Diptera: Culicidae). *J. ent. Soc. sth Afr.*, 24:231–47.

(1965) The environmental background to cases of Burkitt's lymphoma syndrome in Uganda. *E. Afr. med. J.*, 42:62–6.

GREATHEAD, D. J. (1963) A review of the insect enemies of Acridoidea (Orthoptera). *Trans. R. ent. Soc. Lond.*, 114:437–517.

(1966) A brief survey of the effects of biotic factors on populations of the desert locust. *J. appl. Ecol.*, 3:239–50.

(1968) Biological control of *Lantana*—a review and discussion of recent developments in East Africa. *PANS*, 14:167–75.

(1969) On the taxonomy of *Antestiopsis* spp. (Hem., Pentatomidae) of Madagascar, with notes on their biology. *Bull. ent. Res.*, 59:307–315.

GWYNNE, M. D., and BELL, R. H. V. (1968) Selection of vegetation components by grazing ungulates in the Serengeti National Park. *Nature, Lond.*, 220:390–3.

HADDOW, A. J. (1963) An improved map for the study of Burkitt's lymphoma syndrome in Africa. *E. Afr. Med. J.*, 40:429–32.

(1965) Yellow fever in central Uganda, 1964. Part I. Historical introduction. *Trans. R. Soc. trop. Med. Hyg.*, 59:436–40.

HADDOW, A. J., and ELLICE, J. M. (1964) Studies on bush babies (*Galago* spp.) with special reference to the epidemiology of yellow fever. *Trans. R. Soc. trop. Med. Hyg.*, 58:521–38.

HADDOW, A. J., WILLIAMS, M. C., WOODALL, J. P., SIMPSON, D. I. H., and GOMA, L. K. H. (1964) Twelve isolations of Zika virus from *Aedes (Stegomyia) africanus* (Theobald) taken in and above a Uganda forest. *Bull. Wld Hlth Org.*, 31:57–69.

HARLEY, K. L. S., and KUNIMOTO, R. K. (1969) Assessment of the suitability of *Plagiohammus spinipennis* (Thoms.) (Col. Cerambycidae) as an agent for control of weeds of the genus *Lantana* (Verbenaceae). II. Host specificity. *Bull. ent. Res.*, 58:787–92.

HARRIS, W. V. (1961) *Termites, their recognition and control.* Longmans, London.

(1966) Termites and trees: a review of the recent literature. *For. Abstr.*, 27:1–6.

HEDBERG, I., and HEDBERG, O. (eds.) (1968) Conservation of vegetation in Africa south of the Sahara. *Acta Phytogeogr. Suecica*, 54:1–320.

HICKEY, W. A., and CRAIG, G. B. (1966) Distortion of the sex ratio in populations of *Aedes aegypti*. *Can. J. Genet. Cytol.*, 8:260–78.

HODDER, B. W. (1968) *Economic development in the tropics.* Methuen, London.

HOFFMAN, H. A., GOTTLIEB, A. J., and WISECUP, W. G. (1967) Hemoglobin polymorphism in chimpanzees and gibbons. *Science, N.Y.*, 156:944.

HOLLINGSWORTH, M. J., and DUNCAN, C. (1966) The birth weight and survival of Ghanaian twins. *Ann. hum. Genet.*, 30:13–24.

HUFFAKER, C. B. (1959) Biological control of weeds with insects. *A. Rev. Ent.*, 4:251–76.

INGRAM, W. R. (1968) Observations on the control of the coffee berry borer *Hypothenemus hampei* (Ferr.), with endosulfan in Uganda. *Bull. ent. Res.*, 57:539–47.

IRVINE, F. R. (1961) *Woody plants of Ghana with special reference to their uses.* Oxford University Press, London.

ISHIHARA, S. (1964) *Tests for colour blindness.* Lewis, London.

JAGO, N. D. (1968) A checklist of the grasshoppers (Orthoptera, Acrididae) recorded from Ghana, with biological notes and extracts from the literature. *Trans. Am. ent. Soc.*, 94:209–353.

JEFFREYS, M. D. W. (1967) Pre-Columbian maize in southern Africa. *Nature, Lond.*, 215:695–7.

JONES, T. S., and CAVE, A. J. E. (1960) Diet, longevity and dental disease in the Sierra Leone chimpanzee. *Proc. zool. Soc. Lond.*, 135:147–55.

JORDAN, H. D. (1957) Crabs as pests of rice on tidal swamps. *Emp. J. exp. Agric.*, 25:197–206.

JORDAN, P. (1961) *Schistosoma haematobium* infection in a Sukuma village, Tanganyika. *Bull. Wld Hlth Org.*, 25:695–9.

JORDAN, P., and RANDALL, K. (1962) Bilharziasis in Tanganyika: observations on its effects and the effects of treatment in schoolchildren. *J. trop. Med. Hyg.*, 65:1–6.

KATZ, M., and KOPROWSKI, H. (1967) Biological guide to the eradication of communicable diseases: a realistic approach. *Env. Res.*, 1:21–7.

KENNEDY, J. S. (1961) Continuous polymorphism in locusts. In *Insect polymorphism*. Ed. J. S. Kennedy. Royal Entomological Society of London, pp. 80–90.

KNOX, E. G., and MCGREGOR, I. A. (1965) Glucose-6-phosphate dehydrogenase deficiency in a Gambian village. *Trans. R. Soc. trop. Med. Hyg.*, 59:46–58.

KNOX, G., and MORLEY, D. (1960) Twinning in Yoruba women. *J. Obstet. Gynaec. Br. Commonw.*, 67:981–4.

KOCH, A. B. P. W., and LAING, E. (1962) Tuberculosis in Ghana. Mass miniature roentgenographic surveys, 1955–1957. *Am. Rev. resp. Dis.*, 86:159–64.

LAWSON, R. (1963) The economic organization of the *Egeria* fishing industry on the River Volta. *Proc. malac. Soc. Lond.*, 35:273–87.

LEAKEY, L. S. B. (1936) *Kenya contrasts and patterns.* Methuen, London.

LEAN, O. B. (1931) On the recent swarming of *Locusta migratorioides* R. & F. *Bull. ent. Res.*, 22:365–78.

LEEUWANGH, J. (1965) The biology of *Epigynopteryx stictigramma* (Hmps.) (Lepidoptera: Geometridae) a pest of coffee in Kenya. *J. ent. Soc. sth Afr.*, 28:21–31.

LESTON, D. (1970) Entomology of the cocoa farm. *A. Rev. Ent.*, 15:273–94.

LIVINGSTONE, F. B. (1958a) Anthropological implications of the sickle cell gene distribution in West Africa. *Am. Anthropol.*, 60:533–62.

(1958b) The distribution of the sickle cell gene in Liberia. *Am. J. hum. Genet.*, 10:33–41.

(1960) The wave of advance of an advantageous gene: the sickle cell gene in Liberia. *Hum. Biol.*, 32:197–202.

(1961) Balancing the human hemoglobin polymorphism. *Hum. Biol.*, 33:205–19.

(1962) Population genetics and population ecology. *Am. Anthropol.*, 64:44–53.

(1965) The distribution of the abnormal hemoglobin genes and their significance for human evolution. *Evolution, Lancaster, Pa.*, 18:685–99.

LUMSDEN, W. H. R. (1967) Trends in research on the immunology of trypanosomiasis. *Bull. Wld Hlth Org.*, 37:167–75.

MACCUAIG, R. D. (1963) Recent developments in locust control. *Wld Rev. Pest Cont.*, 2:7–17.

MARSDEN, P. D. (1964) The Sukuta project. A longitudinal study of health in Gambian children from birth to 18 months of age. *Trans. R. Soc. trop. Med. Hyg.*, 58:455–89.

MARTIN, P. S. (1966) Africa and Pleistocene overkill. *Nature, Lond.*, 212:339–42.

(1967) Overkill at Olduvai Gorge. *Nature, Lond.*, 215:212–13.

MARTIN, W. J., MORLEY, D., and WOODLAND, M. (1964) Intervals between births in a Nigerian village. *J. trop. Pediatr. Afr. Chld Hlth*, 10:82–5.

MATTINGLY, P. F. (1969) *The biology of mosquito-borne disease*. Allen and Unwin, London.

MCCLELLAND, G. A. H., and WEITZ, B. (1963) Serological identification of the natural hosts of *Aedes aegypti* (L.) and some other mosquitoes (Diptera, Culicidae) caught resting in vegetation in Kenya and Uganda. *Ann. trop. Med. Parasit.*, 57:214–24.

MCGREGOR, I. A. (1960) Demographic effects of malaria with special reference to stable malaria in Africa. *W. Afr. med. J.*, 9:260–5.

(1964) Measles and child mortality in The Gambia. *W. Afr. med. J.*, 13:251–7.

MCGREGOR, I. A., and GILLES, H. M. (1960) Further studies on the control of Bancroftian filariasis in West Africa by means of diethyl-carbamazine. *Ann. trop. Med. Parasit.*, 54:415–18.

MCGREGOR, I. A., RAHMAN, A. K., THOMPSON, B., BILLEWICZ, W. Z., and THOMSON, A. M. (1968) The growth of young children in a Gambian village. *Trans. R. Soc. trop. Med. Hyg.*, 62:341–52.

MCGREGOR, I. A., THOMSON, A. M., and BILLEWICZ, W. Z. (1968) The development of primary teeth in children from a group of Gambian villages, and critical examination of its use for estimating age. *Br. J. Nutr.*, 22:307–14.

MCGREGOR, I. A., WILLIAMS, K., BILLEWICZ, W. Z., and THOMSON, A. M. (1966) Haemoglobin concentration and anaemia in young West African (Gambian) children. *Trans. R. Soc. trop. Med. Hyg.*, 60:650–67.

MCNEIL, M. (1964) Lateritic soils. *Scient. Am.*, 211:96–102.

MEAD, A. R. (1961) *The giant African snail: a problem in economic malacology*. University of Chicago Press, Chicago.

MILLS, A. R. (1967a) The effect of urbanization on health in a mining area of Sierra Leone. *Trans. R. Soc. trop. Med. Hyg.*, 61:114–30.

(1967b) Expatriate personnel in an onchocerciasis endemic region in Sierra Leone. *Trans. R. Soc. trop. Med. Hyg.*, 61:384–9.

MINISTRY OF OVERSEAS DEVELOPMENT (1970) Pest control in rice. *PANS* Manual No. 3.

MIRACLE, M. P. (1966) *Maize in tropical Africa*. University of Wisconsin Press, Milwaukee.
MOREAU, R. E. (1966) *The bird faunas of Africa and its islands*. Academic Press, London.
MOREL, G. (1968) L'impact ecologique de *Quelea quelea* (L.) sur les savanes saheliennes: raisons du pullulement de ce Ploceidae. *Terre Vie*, 1968:69–98.
MORLEY, D. C. (1963) A medical service for children under five years of age in West Africa. *Trans. R. Soc. trop. Med. Hyg.*, 57:79–88.
(1967) Practical approaches to the problems of children in the tropics. *Ind. trop. Hlth*, 6:163–9.
MOTULSKY, A. G., VANDEPITTE, J., and FRASER, G. R. (1966) Population genetic studies in the Congo. 1. Glucose-6-phosphate dehydrogenase deficiency, hemoglobin S, and malaria. *Am. J. hum. Genet.*, 18:514–37.
MULLIGAN, H. W. (ed.) (1971) *The African trypanosomiases*. Allen and Unwin, London.
MURDOCK, G. P. (1959) *Africa—Its people and their culture history*. McGraw-Hill, New York.
(1960) Staple subsistence crops of Africa. *Geogrl Rev.*, 50:521–40.
MUTERE, F. A. (1967) The breeding biology of equatorial vertebrates: reproduction in the fruit bat, *Eidolon helvum*, at latitude 0° 20′ N. *J. Zool., Lond.*, 153:153–61.
NEWSOME, J. (1959) Bilharzia control. *E. Afr. med. J.*, 36:72–5.
NGU, V. A. (1967) The African lymphoma or the Burkitt tumour. *W. Afr. med. J.*, 16:189–97.
NYLANDER, P. P. S. (1971) Ethnic differences in twinning rates in Nigeria. *J. biosoc. Sci.*, 3:151–7.
OTIENO, L. H. (1966) Observations on the action of sisal waste on freshwater pulmonate snails. *E. Afr. agric. For. J.*, 32:68–71.
PIRIE, N. W. (1966) Leaf protein as human food. *Science, N.Y.*, 152:1701–5.
POPLE, W. (1966) Comparison of the *Egeria* fishery of the Sanaga River, Federal Republic of Cameroun with that in the Volta River, Ghana. *Univ. Ghana Volta Basin Res. Proj. Tech. Rep.*, 12:1–4. Mimeographed.
POST, R. H. (1962) Population differences in red and green colour vision deficiency. *Eugen. Q.*, 9:131–46.
PRINGLE, G. (1966) The effect of social factors in reducing the intensity of malaria transmission in coastal East Africa. *Trans. R. Soc. trop. Med. Hyg.*, 60:549–53.
(1969) Experimental malaria control and demography in a rural East African community: a retrospect. *Trans. R. Soc. trop. Med. Hyg.*, 63:2–18.
PRUGININ, Y. (1965) *Report to the Government of Uganda on the experimental fish culture project in Uganda*. Food and Agriculture Organization, Rome.
PURSEGLOVE, J. W. (1968) *Tropical crops. Dicotyledons*. Vols. 1 and 2. Longman, London.
QUENUM, A. (1967) Africa and the problem of contraception. *W. Afr. med. J.*, 16:149–54.

RAYBOULD, J. N. (1968) Change and the transmission of onchocerciasis. *E. Afr. med. J.*, 45:292–4.

ROBERTS, D. F. (1965) Assumption and fact in anthropological genetics. *Jl R. Anthropol. Inst.*, 95:87–103.

(1967) Red/green color blindness in the Niger Delta. *Eugen. Q.*, 14:7–13.

(1969) Race, genetics and growth. *J. biosoc. Sci. Suppl.*, 1:43–67.

ROBERTSON, D. H. H., and BAKER, J. R. (1958) Human trypanosomiasis in south-east Uganda. 1. A study of the epidemiology and present virulence of the disease. *Trans. R. Soc. trop. Med. Hyg.*, 52:337–48.

ROFFEY, J. (1969) The build-up of the present desert locust plague. *PANS*, 15:12–17.

ROFFEY, J., and POPOV, G. (1968) Environmental and behavioural processes in a desert locust outbreak. *Nature, Lond.*, 219:446–50.

ROSEVEAR, D. R. (1969) *The rodents of West Africa*. British Museum (Natural History), London.

RUTISHAUSER, I. H. E. (1962) The food of the Baganda. *Uganda Mus. Occas. Pap.*, 6:1–19.

SAYER, H. J. (1962) The desert locust and tropical convergence. *Nature, Lond.*, 194:330–6.

SCHMUTTERER, H. (1969) *Pests of crops in northeast and central Africa with particular reference to the Sudan*. Fischer, Stuttgart.

SCHWANITZ, F. (1966) *The origin of cultivated plants*. Harvard University Press, Cambridge, Massachusetts.

SIMMONDS, N. W. (1962) *The evolution of bananas*. Longmans, London.

SIMPSON, D. I. H. (1964) Zika virus infection in man. *Trans. R. Soc. trop. Med. Hyg.*, 58:335–8.

SIMPSON, D. I. H., HADDOW, A. J., WILLIAMS, M. C., and WOODALL, J. P. (1965) Yellow fever in central Uganda, 1964. Part IV. Investigations on bloodsucking Diptera and monkeys. *Trans. R. Soc. trop. Med. Hyg.*, 59:449–58.

SMYTH, J. D. (1962) *Introduction to Animal parasitology*. English Universities Press, London.

STAMP, L. D. (1965) *The geography of life and death*. Fontana, London.

STERN, C. (1960) *Principles of human genetics*. Freeman, San Francisco.

STOWER, W. J. (1959) The colour patterns of hoppers of the desert locust. *Anti-Locust Bull.*, 32:1–75.

STOWER, W. J., and GREATHEAD, D. J. (1969) Numerical changes in a population of the desert locust, with special reference to factors responsible for mortality. *J. appl. Ecol.*, 6:203–35.

STURROCK, R. F. (1966) Bilharzia transmission on a new Tanzanian irrigation scheme. *E. Afr. med. J.*, 43:1–6.

SYMMONS, P. M., DEAN, G. J. W., and STORTENBEKER, C. W. (1963) The assessment of the size of populations of adults of the red locust, *Nomadacris septemfasciatus* (Serville), in an outbreak area. *Bull. ent. Res.*, 54:549–69.

TAYLOR, W. (1969) Population prospects for regions of the world. *J. biosoc. Sci. Suppl.*, 1:107–17.

THOMAS, E. M. (1960) *The harmless people*. Secker and Warburg, London.

THOMPSON, B. (1966) The first fourteen days of some West African babies. *Lancet*, 2:40–65.

THOMPSON, B., and RAHMAN, A. K. (1967) Infant feeding and child care in a West African village. *J. trop. Pediatr.*, 13:124–38.

THOMSON, A. M., BILLEWICZ, W. Z., THOMPSON, B., ILLSLEY, R. RAHMAN, A. K., and MCGREGOR, I. A. (1968) A study of growth and health of young children in tropical Africa. *Trans. R. Soc. trop. Med. Hyg.*, 62:330–40.

THOMSON, K. D. B. (1967) Rural health in northern Nigeria: some recent developments and problems. *Trans. R. Soc. trop. Med. Hyg.*, 61:277–302.

TOPLEY, E. (1968a) Common anaemia in rural Gambia. I. Hookworm anaemia among men. *Trans. R. Soc. trop. Med. Hyg.*, 62:579–94.
(1968b) Common anaemia in rural Gambia. II. Iron deficiency anaemia among women. *Trans. R. Soc. trop. Med. Hyg.*, 62:595–601.

TURNBULL, C. (1961) *The forest people.* Simon and Schuster, New York.

UVAROV, B. (1961a) Insect hazards in land development. *Span, Lond.*, 4:154–7.
(1961b) Quantity and quality in insect populations. *Proc. R. ent. Soc. Lond.* C, 25:52–9.
(1964) Problems of insect ecology in developing countries. *J. appl. Ecol.*, 1:159–68.

VESEY-FITZGERALD, D. F. (1963) Central African grasslands. *J. Ecol.*, 51:243–74.

VOLLER, A., and WILSON, H. (1964) Immunological aspects of a population under prophylaxis against malaria. *Br. med. J.*, 2:551–2.

WALOFF, Z. (1962) Flight activity of different phases of the desert locust in relation to plague dynamics. In *Physiologie, comportement et ecologie des acridiens en rapport avec la phase,* CNRS, Paris.

WALSHE, S. L. E., and GILLES, H. M. (1962) Haematological and biochemical observations on a herd of Gambian cattle. *J. comp. Path. Ther.*, 72:439–49.

WARD, P. (1965) Feeding ecology of the black-faced dioch *Quelea quelea* in Nigeria. *Ibis,* 107:173–214.

WATTS, W. S. (1969) Transmission of dieldrin from insects to their offspring. *Nature, Lond.*, 221:762–3.

WEBBE, G., and JORDAN, P. (1966) Recent advances in knowledge of schistosomiasis in East Africa. *Trans. R. Soc. trop. Med. Hyg.*, 60:279–312.

WEGESA, P. (1968) The resettlement of refugees and onchocerciasis in Tanzania. *E. Afr. med. J.*, 45:251–3.

WERNER, G. H., LATTE, B., and CONTINI, A. (1964) Trachoma. *Scient. Am.*, 210:79–86.

WEST, R. (1965) *The white tribes of Africa.* Cape, London.

WHEATLEY, P. E., and CROWE, T. J. (1964) Field studies of insecticides against the coffee leaf-miner *Leucoptera meyricki* Ghesq. (Lepidoptera, Lyonetiidae). *Bull. ent. Res.*, 55:193–203.

WHITEHEAD, P. J. (1960) Interspecific hybrids of *Tilapia: T. nigra* × *T. zillii. Nature, Lond.*, 187:878.

WIESENFELD, S. L. (1967) Sickle-cell trait in human biological and cultural evolution. *Science, N.Y.*, 157:1134–40.

WILLIAMS, C. N., and CASSWELL, G. H. (1959) An insect attacking *Striga. Nature, Lond.*, 184:1668.

WILLIAMS, M. C. (1967) Implications of the geographical distribution of Burkitt's lymphoma. In *Treatment of Burkitt's tumour* ed. J. M. Burchenal and D. Burkitt, Springer, Berlin.

WILLIAMS, M. C., SIMPSON, D. I. H., and SHEPHERD, R. C. (1964) Bats and arboviruses in East Africa. *Nature, Lond.*, 203:670.

WILLIAMS, M. C., and WOODALL, J. P. (1964) An epidemic of an illness resembling dengue in the Morogoro District of Tanganyika. Part II. Virological findings. *E. Afr. med. J.*, 41:271–5.

WILLIAMS, M. C., WOODALL, J. P., CORBET, P. S., and GILLETT, J. D. (1965) O'nyong nyong fever: an epidemic virus disease in East Africa. VIII. Virus isolations from *Anopheles* mosquitoes. *Trans. R. Soc. trop. Med. Hyg.*, 59:300–6.

WILLIAMSON, G., and PAYNE, W. J. A. (1965) *An introduction to animal husbandry in the tropics.* Longmans, London.

WILSON, F. (1964) The biological control of weeds. *A. Rev. Ent.*, 9:225–44.

(1965) Biological control and the genetics of colonizing species. In *The genetics of colonizing species*, Academic Press, New York.

WOODALL, J. P. (1964) The viruses isolated from arthropods at the East African Virus Research Institute in the 26 years ending December 1963. *Proc. E. Afr. Acad.*, 2:141–6.

WOODALL, J. P., and WILLIAMS, M. C. (1967) Tanga virus: a hitherto undescribed virus from *Anopheles* mosquitoes from Tanzania. *E. Afr. med. J.*, 44:83–6.

WOODROW, D. F. (1965) Observations on the red locust (*Nomadacris septemfasciatus* Serv.) in the Rukwa Valley, Tanganyika, during its breeding season. *J. anim. Ecol.*, 34:187–200.

WORLD HEALTH ORGANIZATION (1960) Health aspects of urbanization in Africa. *Wld Hlth Org. Chron.*, 14.

WRIGHT, D. H., BELL, T. M., and WILLIAMS, M. C. (1967) Burkitt's tumour: a review of clinical features, treatment, pathology, epidemiology, entomology and virology. *E. Afr. med. J.*, 44:51–61.

WYNNE-EDWARDS, V. C. (1963) Intergroup selection in the evolution of social systems. *Nature, Lond.*, 200:623–6.

YULE, W. N. (1960) Dieldrin lattices applied by aircraft for controlling hoppers of the red locust, *Nomadacris septemfasciatus* (Serville). *Bull. ent. Res.*, 51:441–60.

INDEX

Pleistocene, 10, 11, 13, 62, 109
Ploceus cucullatus, 102
pneumonia, 39, 44, 171, 194
poliomyelitis, 42
politicians and politics, 15–17, 29, 184
pollution and pollutants, 113, 156, 180–1
polygamy, 15, 25, 36
polymorphism, 162, 168, 170, 171
polytheism, 15
Pople, W., 137–8
Popov, G., 96
population, human, 18, 20–32, 52, 54–5, 63, 64, 142, 147, 148, 160, 163–4, 173–4, 178–82, 187, 188, 191, 198
Portuguese, 13, 14, 65–7, 173–4
Portuguese Guinea, 23, 188, 189
Portulaca, 77
Post, R. H., 170
Pringle, G., 147
Protozoa, 106, 141, 146, 152
Pruginin, Y., 130
Psidium guajava, 76
Purseglove, J. W., 71
pygmies, 9, 12, 13, 49–52, 122, 172
Pyralidae, 101
pyrethrum, 8, 79
Pyrethrum cinerariaefolium, 79
Pyrethrum Marketing Board, 9
Pyricularia oryzae, 100

Queen Elizabeth National Park, 112
Quelea quelea, 98–9, 102
Quenum, A., 22

rabies, 158
Rahman, A. K., 36, 38
rainfall, 2–4, 6, 36, 51, 71, 72, 73, 79, 80, 91, 94, 95, 110, 111, 133, 139
Randall, K., 156, 157
raw materials, *see* resources
Raybould, J. N., 152
Red Sea, 94
relapsing fever, 194
resources, 16, 18–19, 54, 55, 58, 82, 129, 178–83, 186–7
Rhodesia, 23, 182, 188, 189
rice, 37, 56, 71–2, 79–81, 100–3, 196
Ricinus communis, 78
rickets, 131, 173
Rift Valley, 1, 10, 63
rinderpest, 116
road accidents, 56–7
Roberts, D. F., 161, 163, 169, 174, 197, 198
Robertson, D. H. H., 153
rodents, 55, 100, 102–3, 121
Roffey, J., 96, 97
Romanuik, A., 23
Rosevear, D. R., 102
Royal Society of Tropical Medicine and Hygiene, 35, 155
rubber, 82
Rubiaceae, 77
ruff, 102
Rukwa Valley, 92, 111
Rutaceae, 75, 108
Rutishauser, I. H. E., 136
Ruwenzori, 4
Rwanda, 23, 129, 188, 189, 197

Saccharum officinarum, 73
Sahara, 1, 2, 6, 7, 9, 13, 62, 63, 68, 110, 113
Sanaga River, 137–8
Saturniidae, 132
savanna, 1, 3, 4, 5, 6, 7, 10, 16, 36, 48, 62–3, 65, 71, 72, 90, 94, 98, 99, 107, 109, 111–14, 116, 117, 119, 122, 124, 181

Sayer, H. J., 91
scabies, 192
Schistocerca gregaria, 91
Schistosoma haematobium, 153–5, 163, 196; *mansoni*, 153, 156, 157
schistosomiasis, 153–7, 194, 197
Schmutterer, H., 104
Schwanitz, F., 64
Scolytidae, 105
seasons (wet and dry), 1–3, 36–8, 40, 41, 42, 45, 72, 76, 79–81, 111, 112, 133, 145, 190
Senegal, 48, 49, 99, 188, 189
Senegal River, 10
Serengeti National Park, 113–14
sesame, 88
Sesamum indicum, 88
Sesarma huzardi, 101
sex ratio, in man, 24–5, 31–2, 191; in mosquitoes, 144
sheep, 119, 120–1
Shepherd, R. C., 150
Sherbro, 191
shifting cultivation, 69
Shilluk, 174, 197, 198
shrimps, 101
sickle cell, 140, 148, 164–9
Sierra Leone, 3, 4, 24, 28–32, 35, 53, 54, 56, 59–61, 77, 79–81, 101, 102, 107, 128, 129, 138, 142, 179, 185, 188, 189, 191, 194
Simmonds, N. W., 75
Simpson, D. I. H., 149, 150, 151
Simulium, 61, 152; *damnosum*, 152
sisal, 78, 156
skin colour, 172–3
sleeping sickness, 152–3
smallpox, 142, 157, 172
Smith, A., 144
Smyth, J. D., 146
snails, 37, 50, 55, 101, 108, 137, 145; aquatic, 153–6
snakes, 121
soil, 4, 6
Solanaceae, 77, 78
Solanum melongena, 77
Somali Republic and peninsula, 23, 94, 97, 188
sorghum, 36, 63, 67, 71, 72, 78, 85
Sorghum vulgare, 71
South Africa, 16, 91, 116
Spaniards, 174
Spodoptera exempta, 13, 98
Stamp, L. D., 123, 141
stem-borers, 80, 101
Sterculiaceae, 78
Stern, C., 140
stork, Abdim's, 134
Stortenbeker, C. W., 93
Stower, W. J., 96, 97
Striga, 87
Sturrock, R. F., 154
Sudan, 12, 15, 23, 48, 188, 189
sugar cane, 73
Sukuma, 155
Sukuta (The Gambia), 39–41, 192
Sus scrofa, 121; *vittatus*, 121
Susu, 191
Swahili, 12, 173
sweet potato, 74, 80
Symmons, P. M., 93

tangerine, 75
Tanzania and Tanganyika, 12, 69, 95, 111, 113–14, 129, 150, 152, 155, 156, 188, 189, 196, 197
Taylor, W., 198

B5